Binge Eating

A Self-help Guide to Recovery From Eating Disorder

(How to Stop Binge Eating Fast Whilst Still Enjoying Your Free Time)

Angela Hensley

Published By **Ryan Princeton**

Angela Hensley

All Rights Reserved

Binge Eating: A Self-help Guide to Recovery From Eating Disorder (How to Stop Binge Eating Fast Whilst Still Enjoying Your Free Time)

ISBN 978-1-77485-973-5

No part of this guidebook shall be reproduced in any form without permission in writing from the publisher except in the case of brief quotations embodied in critical articles or reviews.

Legal & Disclaimer

The information contained in this ebook is not designed to replace or take the place of any form of medicine or professional medical advice. The information in this ebook has been provided for educational & entertainment purposes only.

The information contained in this book has been compiled from sources deemed reliable, and it is accurate to the best of the Author's knowledge; however, the Author cannot guarantee its accuracy and validity and cannot be held liable for any errors or omissions. Changes are periodically made to this book. You must consult your doctor or get professional medical advice before using any of the suggested remedies, techniques, or information in this book.

Upon using the information contained in this book, you agree to hold harmless the Author from and against any damages, costs, and expenses, including any legal fees potentially resulting from the application of any of the information provided by this guide. This disclaimer applies to any damages or injury caused by the use and application, whether directly or indirectly, of any advice or information presented, whether for breach of contract, tort, negligence, personal injury, criminal intent, or under any other cause of action.

You agree to accept all risks of using the information presented inside this book. You need to consult a professional medical practitioner in order to ensure you are both able and healthy enough to participate in this program.

Table Of Contents

Chapter 1: An Adventure Down Memory Lane 1

Chapter 2: A Larger Look At Our Habitual Patterns 25

Chapter 3: Happiness Effect 59

Chapter 4: The Future Path 88

Chapter 5: Mindfulness Is The Key 112

Chapter 6: What Is Binge Eating Disorder And How Can It Be Treated? 135

Chapter 7: What Signs And Symptoms Are Possible In Binge Eating 143

Chapter 8: The Complications Binge-Eating People Can Expect 147

Chapter 9: What Psychotherapy Treatments, & Medications Would Work? 152

Chapter 10: A Healthy Regimen With A Good Support Group 161

Chapter 11: The Self-Management Strategies That Will Help You Take Control 178

Chapter 1: An Adventure Down Memory Lane

It may seem scary to face your demons, but let's not forget that we've already done the right thing. This is very brave. When we first realize something is needed, it opens the door for us to explore the unknown. It's going to get easier from here, which is the good news. There will always be doubts, but they will disappear as we progress. It doesn't matter whether you eat to get bored or to alleviate stress. . This is how dangerous things can become. You just know that eating gives you some form of comfort or relief. The downward spiral is already underway.

Eating to deal with our emotions is a regular habit. It would be normal to exercise every single day, for example.

It's not something you would think twice about. This holds true for any habit or routine, no matter how positive or negative. If it's negative, it can be dangerous. It becomes dangerous if emotional eating is a part of our daily routine. It will quickly become a habitual behavior that we don't even think about. As humans, we depend on our routines. They are absolutely essential. They become second nature once they become part of our daily routines. It's not that you are lazy or incapable of self-control. The best thing about this knowledge is that we can adapt and change our routines. Any moment can be used to make changes in our lives, and habits are no exception. As you can see you're not far away. Only because you are a regular eater, your path to despair has become a habit.

Self-Reflection: A Hawk's View

Knowing that our emotional eating patterns have become a habit, it's time for us to take a step back and reflect. This is where you will dig into the root causes of your eating habits. Can you think of a time you only ate for the sake of eating? Or are you simply observing? Does eating seem more like going back to the pantry multiple times? Retrospectively, we might be able to see things differently than we did at the time. Our actions can be viewed through a fine lens. It's almost like seeing our own behavior from the eyes of a hawk. One example is a hawk flying high above town and seeing everything. He would see everything: cars, people and buildings. He would be able to see things in a way that no one else can. This will allow us to tackle the most important issues. It will give you an advantage. You'll see everything as it really is. We can step back and examine when things started to go wrong. Is it the first time that you reached for a candybar even though you weren't hungry. Did it happen when you ate way more than you ought to at dinner? While it may not seem like much at first, these little things are what caused problems. Doing these little things every day will make them a daily habit. It may seem as though we have only eaten a single candy bar once or overindulged in pasta salad. Like any habitual behaviour, eating is not an exception. There are other things you could have done, instead of eating the candy bars. This may have been an innocent way to deal with the situation. It is not a matter of satiating our cravings with candy bars, but rather filling the time. It doesn't matter whether we're bored or just feeling unoccupied. It is an excuse that allows us to fill this time.

While we might think that we are trying to curb appetite, are we really eating for our health? Did your stomach start to churn? Even if your stomach was grumbling, it is not common for us to eat candy bars as a meal.

If you view these things from a hawks' perspective, you will see how they add up. Understanding the development of emotional eating habits is key to addressing our core problems and getting to the root cause of the problem. While they may seem like small steps, they have a big impact on the overall picture. All these little actions add up over time to make our routines. Soon enough it becomes a habitual occurrence, and soon we are scavenging the pantry without good reasons. As you can see you are not at fault for things going south. It is simply human nature. We are creatures of habit. While it may be that you are simply bored, some people have deeper connections to unhealthy eating habits. For instance, we may find that we eat more often when we feel stressed. It is possible that we do not understand why we eat. We just know it provides some relief. There is no other reason than to get a brief relief. As I said, you don't need to be harsh about yourself. Let's take a step back and look at ourselves from an objective viewpoint. If it makes you feel less harsh about yourself, you can continue to adopt the hawks' stance. Keep in mind that you are not the only person doing this. You are taking important steps toward becoming your best self.

Moving forward from heartache and turmoil will require that we understand the roots of our pain. Reflection on our past can give us a new perspective. Without self-reflection, it would be difficult to continue the same path as before. If we want change to occur, it is important to identify the issues that need to change. I encourage you to take a moment and reflect on what you are doing. Start by asking yourself if your eating habits are due to boredom, stress, or both. No matter the emotion trigger, put it there. Is it boredom that causes you to eat? Are you taking a break during your day? Maybe it is evening or night. Take a look at your environment at the time. Once we have an idea of what is causing our eating patterns, we can implement changes. It's the same for feelings of anxiety or stress. Whatever emotion is causing your need for comfort food, we're going to address it. Find the part of your day that makes you feel stressed. You might feel stressed at lunch, just before peak business hours. You might feel stressed or anxious about the remainder of your day. This is normal. A snack would help relieve the stress. This could also be related to bored eating. Maybe you eat more at night because you feel like it fills a void. Or maybe you are trying to reduce stress. This is important to consider, regardless of the situation. You have a responsibility to recognize the causes of your emotional eating. No matter what circumstance, we turn to food to ease our pain.

Addressing the Core Problems

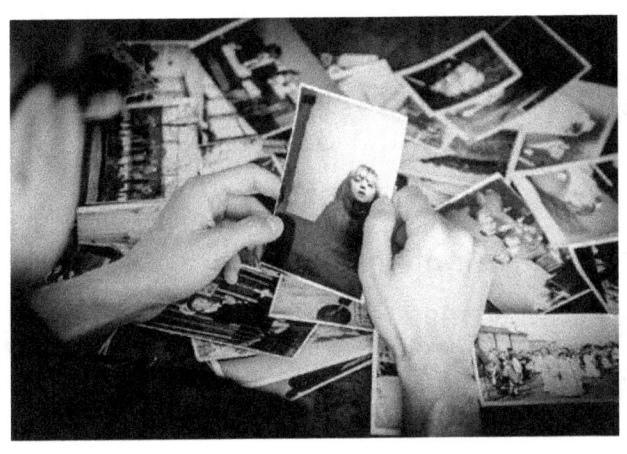

Once we understand where our eating habits are coming from, we can then begin to heal it. We must not use the hawks' perspective to observe our eating habits or actions. This is a different way of healing. We must first identify what is causing these negative emotions. We can heal by using a magnifying mirror. The magnifying glasses allow you to examine every corner, crevice, and curve. You can see things you couldn't otherwise see. The same is true for healing our negative emotions. We will look at the thoughts and emotions behind them. To do that, you will need to place your magnifying lens over any thoughts you have before you eat. What thoughts are going through our minds just before we start to eat? We may share a few things in common with our minds when it comes down to the mind. This could be, for instance, repeating the one mistake you made over a number of times. The constant thought of it makes you wish things were different. As if we could somehow create a magical time machine to bring it back. This isn't possible. However, we all come up with situations or linger over things that don't deserve our time. All of these actions can contribute towards emotional eating. Unfortunately, we all fall for these thoughts. With a fine lens we can examine our thoughts and identify what is causing our emotional eating. We can better understand our thoughts by looking at them. Boredom will often act as a defense mechanism for thoughts and feelings that aren't really appealing to you. Eating can help us to avoid these feelings and thoughts, rather than allowing them to become more real.

Let's stop consuming food to combat these negative thoughts. This is a simple way to fix negative thoughts or feelings. In reality, we are the causes of our own suffering. You may have heard similar statements. But it is true. Our thoughts influence our emotions, and we are actually the creators of those thoughts. We believe that something is causing us to be angry or upset. Someone cut your traffic lane, and you're now mad. It's easy to think that traffic has caused you anger. While this can be frustrating, it is not the actual cause of our anger. This can be a trigger or external source of anger. Also, we can take a step back from this and see that it is only us who are clinging on to the source of our pain. We can choose to observe this irritation and not get angry. You can then shift your focus to the idea that these are temporary events. The pain and anger you feel does not have to be endured. You shouldn't be critical about your past mistakes or failures. By clinging to these thoughts, we only cause ourselves pain. There are some things that we can do to combat these negative emotions. To be objective, as in the traffic situation, is the first. The second is to be more objective and see yourself from a bird's-eye view. Instead of feeling angry, you can instead observe anger and realize that it is just an emotion. It is not you. It is something that will flow through your body and you can let it go. Self-compassion is another technique for dealing with emotions. You can tell you many things to help make you feel better. It is possible to tell yourself that nothing can stop you. Even if you are feeling overwhelmed, you can get through it. A journal is a great way to track negative emotions. We will be less inclined to rely on food for comfort once we have learned that we can heal ourselves. Instead, we can find our own inner peace.

It is crucial to understand the root cause of our thoughts, emotions, environment, and how they affect us. However, we must also look at what boredom can mean for us. Why do you eat more when bored? Do you want to be entertained or do you feel impatient? Like we have the power to let our thoughts and emotions flow, so too can we choose not to feel bored. Boredom can be overcome by finding something to replace it. We have the option to choose not to feel bored.

Finding something to entertain ourselves can help us get rid of this feeling. If you find yourself looking for something to distract you, such as a snack or a pantry item to grab, it is likely that you have already found what you need. Instead of resorting to eating to satisfy this void, there are several things we can do. Although eating seems like the obvious choice, it's also the most natural thing to do. When we are constantly eating useless snacks, it can become very difficult to eat. It may seem like snack after snack depending on how busy we are. This could lead us to overeaten. Because this is part of our daily routine, we don't realize how badly it may be affecting them. This could lead to serious health problems. It can cause us to eat out of boredom all the time, and we don't pay attention to how many calories we are eating. Sometimes we eat because we're bored. It doesn't matter if you are eating out of boredom or stress. We can ask the same questions. What is the cause of this stress? You can find a better way of coping by understanding why you are stressed. Our first instinct might be to turn to food as it offers some relief. However, this is not the right way to deal with stress. It is important to feel the feelings you have so that we can understand why they are stressing. If this does not help, there are healthy ways to manage stress. Music can be soothing if you like to listen to music even when you are sad. There are many methods to reduce stress but going to the pantry is not an effective option. We want to avoid these feelings when they arise. Music can be soothing, but exercise is also an option. It seems that exercise of any kind can relieve the stress from the mind, which sometimes is hard to put out.

While I don't know how dire your situation has become, let us recall a time when we weren't bored with food. Was there anything you were doing when you had the time? What are some fun things that you can do to pass the day? Do you have any hobbies that can pass the time? A walk in the park, or an evening fishing trip are good alternatives. These are all healthy ways to keep busy, and not just to unconsciously decide to eat. We eat when we are bored. It's an unconscious act. We don't actively think about what we could do with our time. It seems almost as though we just want what they are craving. These seemingly mindless acts result in a new habit.

To stop eating bored food, it is important to first recall our old habits. They are the productive ones. Remember how you felt active in their creation. This is probably good. We felt satisfied and happy. These positive emotions can vary depending upon what your hobby is. If you love reading, for instance, you may feel calmer and more at ease. While someone who enjoys reading can feel relaxed and content, someone who works out at the gym could feel accomplished and confident. These feelings can be associated with productivity, no matter what the activity. These small habits are more productive than bored eating. This is a mindless, ineffective activity that eventually leads to even more negative results. It is easy to see why this behavior can lead to a downward spiral. We can change this behavior, as with any other habit. You can stop boring eating by making it a habit. Which was your hobby before everything went wrong? What was your first hobby? Let's get to the bottom of it. Keep a journal to remember your particular hobby. It is important to understand why and how we want to change our habits. It is possible to recall positive emotions that are associated with old habits and envision how they can positively benefit our lives. Keep a journal to reflect on your feelings and old hobbies. For clarity, recall any details you'd like to know about your hobby. Keep track of the outfits you wore to the gym or what fishing gear you used to like to fish with. Knowing everything about your past hobbies can help you feel more connected. These hobbies will eventually end. These hobbies can be reconnected or even formed new ones to help with boredom. It's possible to find new hobbies by researching similar interests to those you already have. If you're someone who loves going to the gym, it might be worth looking at a different workout routine. It doesn't matter what hobby you are passionate about, this will work well for you. It should feel exciting. It's possible to forget why you started eating in the first instance. Hobbies are a great way to add some joy and "me time" into your life. You won't even wish you were eating... except maybe for a slice of pizza once in a while. This will not be the same as eating unconsciously for no reason.

It is easy to see how a positive habit like going for a walk or to the gym can be a learned one. It could be that someone taught us about going to the fitness center. Perhaps a friend goes to the gym, and we decide to start working out there. Or maybe we went to the gym and saw it firsthand, which led us into signing up. It didn't matter what way we looked, we found the habit of going the gym and began to do it. This is how we came across the hobby. How did this become a hobby? The gym could have been something that a family member or friend introduced us to. We could have done it all on our own. You might want to think about how you learned this habit. Is it something you learned from your family? You could just eat what they served. Perhaps you would have eaten a whole bag full of popcorn if you were seated to watch a film. You can pass your habits on to the people you surround yourself with, especially if these are your parents. Yes, it can even be related to what we eat. You might find people around you who enjoy eating out a lot. You might be like others who only eat out for special occasions. There are many possible explanations for your unhealthy eating habits. You can choose which one to follow. These are some things that you can add to your diary.

Like we said, we can eat in a few minutes or go out to eat. Boredom eating is also possible when you go out for food. There are many temptations to eat unhealthy food at restaurants or consume more food. If you make it a regular event, rather than just a once in a while occasion, you will be creating a pattern. You won't feel great if you eat the same foods every time we go out for dinner or just randomly visit the pantry. It is possible to feel tired and hungry when we are not eating as much. The same could happen when eating out. You'll be adding unhealthy foods to your diet. This can lead to conflict later. As with the choice to eat out, choosing a healthy option can be a decision.

I will briefly refer to the quote that was mentioned at the start of the book. It states that "Eat your body to fuel your soul." We must also eat healthy food choices. Our body needs to be fed high-quality food. Not quantity. For example, adding healthy foods into our diet will give us the energy that we need to keep healthy. All foods can be added, including vegetables, fruits (including dairy), healthy fats, oil, and meat. We can also make certain foods, such as junk food, and avoid processed foods. You can even reduce or eliminate soda and alcohol by drinking more water. Not only will this help us adopt healthier eating habits, but it will also allow us to eat more healthy foods. It is important to consider what foods you love eating in order for you to choose the best option. Paleo is a diet that allows you to eat fish and not meat. There are many choices when it comes to food. You can research your options or hire a professional lifestyle coach or dietician to help guide you. It will make a difference in our lives and help to decrease emotional eating. Energy is more important when we eat healthy. Energy can make us feel happier, and give us more energy to be productive.

You are still here. All of these steps have been taken forward and I am prouder than ever of you. It can be hard to start our own journey. You have already made great strides on your journey and are now ready to face the more difficult parts of your story. That takes courage, guts, and courage. We now know where it began to get dark. It is easy to see the downfall when we fly above it all. It is interesting to look back on how our lives have changed from just eating to what we are today. This is how it will be at end of the journey. It will all be worth it when you look back in the future. This was the spark that ignited it. You are about be a full-blown phoenix. It's a transformation you never dreamed possible, and I am so excited for your success. It is happening now. It's all in the planning. All of the knowledge that we now have will make it easier for us to move. We'll be able to go back to where things were. Not only that, but they will be even more successful than they were before. In fact, it may even be ten times better. Remember, even though we might be looking back, this journey will propel us forward into our new way.

Chapter 2: A Larger Look At Our Habitual Patterns

Once we have an understanding of who we are and how we got here we can start to see how our habits develop. It is very easy to make a habit that you don't even know is there. This is why we're not responsible for it. We all fall prey to it. Our habits are a result of our habitual nature. If we don't pay attention, we can easily fall into negative patterns. Once we are aware of a bad habit, it's possible to make changes. It may not be easy to change this habitual eating behavior, but it can be done. It is clear that you don't have to change. Our habitual nature can be seen as normal and part in human life. This will help us feel more empowered. We need to have habits in order to be successful in our lives. They are our foundation for security and comfort. They are stored in the subconscious mind and become part our daily life. The habit of eating is a natural part of our lives. One day we find ourselves unable to stop eating. We end up wondering how and why this happened. We unconsciously created a pattern out of our food. Unconsciously, this behaviour became a regular part of our daily lives. This became a common way to find comfort and food, and soon became a routine.

Habits and Their Purposes

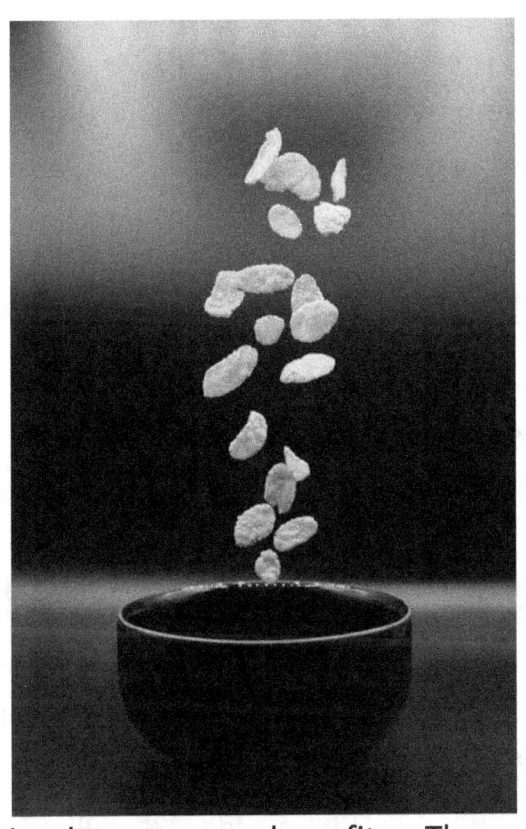

Habits have many benefits. They can provide stability and allow us to work efficiently. Habits help us live more productive lives. When we go shopping, we know what we want, because we have a tendency to buy the same things. We tend to buy the same hair products and makeup as we do food. If we had to search for a new list each time, it would consume a lot more time and energy. It is not an ingrained habit to get the same products. This holds true for activities such as brushing teeth or getting up each morning to make our beds. Each person makes their bed in a unique way. How many pillows should I use? How do we fold our blankets, and how do we tuck in our bed sheets? Each person's method is different, but it is the best. It is our daily routine. Even if we do not make our bed every day for a few days, it will remain a part of our daily routine. Although we may make it once a day, we will still be able to use the same spot for pillows. We crave stability so we fall into routines. We like to know what foods we are going to eat and how to make our beds. The conservation of energy is another way that habits can be beneficial. As I mentioned, if you had to come up with a new grocery shopping list with different items each time you went to the supermarket, it would be exhausting. Habits can be unconsciously created and maintained so that we can conserve energy and perform tasks as if there is no need to think. This allows us not only to be efficient but also to have more brain power for other tasks.

You may be unconscious when you reach for something sweet or go to the grocery store. You can be unconscious if you reach for a bag full of chips at a specific time each day. These actions are not conscious. It's something we do. We can get up and run to the fridge, without even having to do anything. We know this activity is relaxing. This activity brings stability to our day, so it is just a regular thing for us. Sometimes, however, we don't realize the consequences of our habits over time. We eventually reach our limit. You suddenly realize your habits may need to be adjusted. Hopefully we will see this before it becomes too late. Sometimes, however, we reach a point when we're fed up and want to change. But how can this be done? What can we do to stop this habit from becoming a permanent fixture in our lives? Here's how. All that is required is your desire to change. You've already made that change and are continuing to do so. If you are determined to make positive changes, it is possible to start a snowball effect. You can build momentum, and then tumble to the finish line feeling free from your unhealthy eating.

Falling into Comfort

We are all creatures of habits so you have an advantage when it comes to changing our lives. It is not your fault for the way you eat, which should be comforting. The fact that you aren't entirely responsible can relieve some of the pressure. You might feel ready to begin your race, and that you are worthy of this change. Let's start by understanding what it means to have a habitual nature. Habitual patterns could include brushing your teeth and applying your makeup. These are all things that can be done without conscious thought. It's as if the steps are all laid out and we only have to follow them. You brush your own teeth every morning. It's something you do every day. It's not something we do with conscious effort. It's easy to just do our routine and stand there while we brush our teeth. These are the things which give us the feeling of more stability. We want and need stability. It doesn't matter if you are making your morning cup of coffee, or sitting down to read the paper at the breakfast table. We all need our stability. You have comfort and stability no matter how bad it may be for your life. You are faced with these two things like a bull in the head. If you lack the tools to take on these challenges and change your behaviour, you will not be able do so. We as humans need stability and comfort. That is the whole purpose of our habits. It can be hard to break a negative habit. It's possible. It's not impossible, just as it is with everything. Everything we do has a significant impact on us. Positive mindsets can greatly help us win and be victorious. It is easy to form and keep good habits. But it can be so difficult to break these bad habits. We are drawn to our comfort areas. Anything outside of those comfort zones seems like work. You don't just like your comfort zone, but you also have to break a habit. This can be quite strange when we try to change a bad habit. We became so used to this way of living. Habits aren't just actions and behaviours, but an integral part of our lives. They are almost part of our identity. We are all familiar with how we brush our teeth. They provide structure to our lives. It's just different without them. If we can get rid off a negative habit and replace it by something better, it will have positive effects on the rest of our lives. It could even change our lives. Imagine how a positive habit can improve your quality of life. Think about how these positive habits can be associated with you. Your life will improve dramatically.

Habits vs. Routines

What does a "habit" mean if we are habitual creatures? What does it mean to have habits and what do they contribute to our nature? Habits like humans are made up of a variety of components. Habits, like humans, are created through a psychological pattern called the habit loop. It includes three components: the cue (or routine), the reward (or reward). The cue is any thing that encourages you to do a habit. You can use the cue to indicate your mood, place, time, activity, or emotional state. For instance, you might visit the fridge at a particular time each night. Your cue would be night time. The cue is followed by routine. Routine is actually the actual behavior. In this example, it's simply the act of going into the fridge, buying food and eating it. Finally, the reward. When you participate in a behavior, the reward is what makes it a habit. It is the positive reinforcement offered with every habit. It could be the little piece of cheese that you get from the fridge, or the feeling of emotional fulfillment. We must be aware of our habits and how they affect us. It is essential to be aware how our habits affect us. To break the cycle of negative habits and avoid getting stuck in them again, it is a good idea to reward yourself. Consider the benefits of quitting drinking. Do you think it would improve your overall mood? If this is the case, then you can start to change your daily routine and pay more attention about your emotional state.

Knowing that we are creatures habitual, we need to examine our habits and learn more about them. There is a distinction. Habits refer to the unconsciously done things that are automatic and do not require conscious effort. Routines require conscious effort. Routines can be defined as things we want to do. Changes to, additions to, or removals to a routine require that we actually desire to do them. This is where the difference is, and it can be tricky. We might let ourselves down or lose our routines which makes it more difficult to change something in our lives. Let's suppose we want to go the gym every day at a given time. We decided that Monday was a better day to go than Monday. This could cause some disruption to our routine, as our goal was for us to go at a certain time. The next day, however, you decided to stop going. This led to yet another day of not going to the gym. Gradually, we started to fall out of our routine more often. We decided to change our routine. It might seem harder to get back on track if you make changes. You might decide you don't want go. These decisions can be made consciously.

Effectively making a new routine a daily habit is vital. You cannot let yourself slip during this process. Sometimes we may feel it doesn't make a difference to go to work early or stay up late to exercise. It does matter if your goal is to get to the gym at certain times. It doesn't matter if it doesn't, so we send the message to ourselves that it is okay for us to do it again. We won't be as strict, which means that we will not reach our goal. Most effective would be to choose a time to go to the gym every morning and then just do it at that time. This will ensure that it becomes a daily part of your routine. You will find that it doesn't seem strict, but you are just doing your regular day.

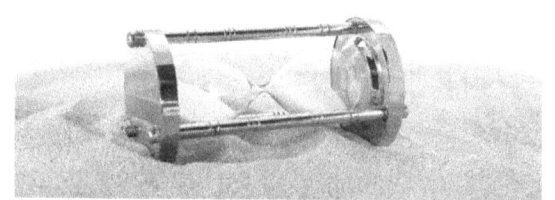

This requires us to put in more effort. But, you can change or implement any routine at any time. All you have to do to keep your mind focused is to make it happen. One way to make a negative habit more productive is to change it. You might try adding more activity to your daily routine, such as walking, if you are a more passive person. Whatever the changes, consistency is important when you are changing your routine. Our routines may become more like habits over time. When we participate in them so frequently, it becomes more unconscious than conscious. This is why some people like to vary their routines. You might consider adding a different type of workout to your day if you already go to the gym almost every day. It might be enough to just change the muscle groups you usually work on each day. There is very little flexibility when making it less routine. It's already a routine. You can just add or remove small things without changing the whole thing.

It's possible to turn routines into habits. Routines like going to school are one example of routines that can eventually become a pattern. If we regularly go to school every day, then it is very likely that the majority of our routines will eventually become a part of our daily life. It is easy to become accustomed to things such as taking the bus, going to school every day, and even studying right after school. These are things that we do every day without even realizing it. They are so normal that it is just a natural thing for us to do. We don't need think about what lunch will look like at school. We go to the cafeteria, place our bags on the ground, and start walking towards the lunch line. We wait in the line, make eye contact with the lunch ladies, and then get our food. We decide what beverage we want and go to the cashier. We pay for the lunch, have a chat with the cashier, and then return to our tables. These are all things we do unconsciously. These are all routines that are part of our daily life. This allows the mind to be consciously focused on different food options, other people, or what drink we will choose at end of line. Habits allow life to flow smoothly when they become routines. We must follow our routines daily, so it's easy to make them automatic. Our attention can be focused elsewhere. It is because teachers don't put a test on us when we first start school. Although there is much material to learn and a lot to do, the students still need to adapt to the new routines. The same applies to our classes. As a result, many basic tasks will become familiar. Thanks to habits, we are blessed. We would certainly not be able to focus our attention on every aspect of our day.

It is not surprising to learn that people tend to be comfortable with what they are familiar with. It can be very difficult to break out of a comfort zone once it is established. We want to believe we can achieve our dreams so that we are less likely question the things that satisfy us. Our only certainty is that we are satisfied. Our brain will not stop pursuing our dreams if they aren't fulfilled. Only when we are unhappy will we decide to make a difference. After we notice that we have gained weight, eating can be a comfortable habit. We are more likely than not to notice the change and will want to make it happen. It will not be easy to abandon the familiar. Once we start to work, however, it will be much more manageable than it might seem. The results will be more satisfying once you make a conscious effort at changing your routines. We won't eat just to satisfy our wants, but will implement a new method to satisfy this hunger. The new way of living can satisfy our desires and replace the old ways that have led to unwanted weight gain. As habitual creatures by nature we will become habitual to positive routines in no time.

Next time you feel like your life is out of control, that's a sign it might be time to change some routines. Changes in behavior can make all the difference if you are feeling low or constantly feel sad. The way we feel can be affected greatly by our habits and routines. These routines can have a positive or negative impact on our lives. Imagine feeling more sluggish or depressed. It's hard to explain why but you know that you have been too busy and don't have the time to cook. Because you aren't eating healthy, most nights you order take-out and fast food. These are habits we have cultivated in our lives. Although it may seem like an unconscious decision to stop for food on the road home, it is actually a habit. This may not be obvious at the time, but it can have a serious impact on our lives. We only know that we're hungry and do not have enough time to make dinner. While there are many options, we often just say we don't have enough time. While it may seem to offer the most reward, it can actually be detrimental to our mental health. As we feel more lazy, we might stop working out as much. This could lead to us making excuses for the behavior that is not working for us. This could be you. This is a great moment to be more aware. You can take a step back and examine all of your actions, allowing you to see things from the perspective of a hawk. With the hawk's eyes, we can see that all of these factors may be contributing to why we feel this way. Instead of feeling stuck, you can take control and make changes.

It's time to break old habits

It is important to reflect on how long it has been a habit before changing them. You might find it helpful to think back to when these habits began. This will give an indication of the difficulty it will be to get rid of our old habits. The more we keep our habits, the harder it is to break them. Because we love to be comfortable and feel safe, the longer we keep them in place the more we will retain those comforts. This goes beyond habits. It could be that your friends are like your comfort zone if they have been around since childhood. Your childhood friends could be like a security blanket. They can offer support and help you feel more stable in this world. You may come to a place in your life when you realize that you've matured. You may be able to see the truth about yourself and want to change it, but this old blanket is keeping you from doing so. You don't know where you should start. And, quite honestly, it is hard to imagine yourself as close to anyone new. This holds true for the long-established habits that we have. Sometimes we may not know where or how to start. This is because we have become so attached and secure with this security blanket it will be very difficult for us to change. Because of how familiar we have become with these habits, it will be much harder to break them. We humans aren't meant to change everything. Our peace of heart is found in our routines, habits and routines. There is still hope, regardless of how old your habits. There are always options to improve our lives.

Changes in life can be difficult at first. What can help us to stay calm is the long-term view. In our case we're deciding to change our eating habits and create a healthier lifestyle. It will make our lifestyle more positive and improve our overall outlook. Although it might seem daunting and intimidating, this transformation will prove to be worthwhile in the long-term. This information will help us to shift our habits to healthier ones. It might seem like things are getting more scary. This is probably a positive thing. This indicates that we are on the brink of something. It means that as we begin to learn this, we move closer to living our dream lives. The easier it is to let go old habits, the more we move forward in forming new habits. It is possible to feel overwhelmed at first.

These are some of the things to remember as you try to get rid of an old habit. Before we can stay committed to the change we want, we need to understand why. It is possible that we will feel uncomfortable, as our old habits are a source of stability. This can increase our feeling of overwhelming. Sometimes we feel like a fish without water. This is normal when we are making changes to our lives. It is possible to find some comfort by reminding oneself of their "why." This helps us remember why we wanted this change. Recalling our why can allow us to move forward without wanting back to our old ways.

Once we have made the decision to make a change in our lives, it is now time to end our old habits. First, we need to recognize our routine. What we really want to eliminate is the routine. To change our routine, for example, we can wake up earlier and stop sleeping late. You might try setting an alarm or going to bed earlier. Once we have established the routine, we can now shift our focus towards the rewards. Rewards are usually the reason our habits develop in the first place. Our actions are often followed by positive rewards that encourage us to keep doing the same behavior. You might find a few benefits when you sleep in. One way to increase our sleep quality is to sleep in, which can help us feel more rested and less cold. When we change our habits, however, we have different options. We can limit how much sleep we get instead of going crazy with our sleeping habits. So we don't lose any time and arrive on time at work. Alternately, we can choose to go bed earlier to allow for more sleep. Once we know our reward, it is time to start looking at our triggers. This will help us navigate through them better in the future. Our triggers are what prompts us to perform the action. You might want to change your alarm if you are one of those people who sleeps in after your alarm clock goes off. It might be possible to move the alarm clock so that it wakes us up. Instead of falling back asleep, you will need to walk over and turn the clock off. If we are able to identify the components of our habit loops, then we can ensure that they do not happen on repeat. You can easily change your routine by making small adjustments and understanding why these habits have developed.

Sometimes, it is possible to run into some problems when we are trying to change our own habits. Habits can be easily created, but they are usually not easy to break. Again, no shame to you. You may have tried a few times to eliminate your bad habits and failed. This is normal. Habits can be hard to change. They have a negative reward and can be hard to break. But this should not discourage anyone. Instead, this can be an empowering sign that we are able to change. The minor problems we might encounter along the journey are nothing major. Each setback we overcome can show us that we're getting stronger. We will soon be at the top looking down at how far our climb has gone. We must begin our climb by adding all the necessary tools to help us reach our goal.

Conditioning is the first thing that can be used to your advantage. This fits in well with a positive mentality. Or, what helps us feel good and move forward. Maybe you can take a look at what thoughts are influencing your eating habits. This can help us get rid of the eating habit we created earlier. You can tackle the problem head-on if you notice that eating is often associated with negative thoughts or feelings. This will make it so much easier to change our routine. This is part our conditioning. It is possible for habits to form in our memory systems when we have a tendency to think or feel a certain manner for extended periods. These negative feelings can be part of your habits. It isn't just what you eat, it's your negative thoughts. These have become habits. Self-help tools could be another way to combat this bad habit. A guidebook or motivational podcast might help us to overcome our emotional eating. Accountability and incentives can be a powerful tool. When we hold ourselves accountable, we are committed to achieving a goal and are likely to be successful--especially when that goal involves being committed to someone else. You might consider sharing your goal with close friends and family to help you be more accountable. In turn, this will make it more likely that you achieve your goals. To make it more motivating, you can offer yourself an incentive. One example of an incentive to lose weight is the image of yourself as someone who has lost their entire weight. It should be what motivates you and makes it possible to hold yourself accountable at night.

These tools will allow us to reach our goals. First, you must resolve to change your life. You are already well on your way. Many people don't recognize the need for change. They live their lives as they are, without realizing that they have the power to make changes in their lives. If something is not right about us, we can change it. Our habits make up our lives. We depend on them for security and can even identify with them. Because they are all made up our own behavior, they reflect who we really are. If we have unhealthy or negative habits, then we could be called unhealthy. This is not something we want to hear, but it is true. It is possible to change a habit at any time. Even though we may identify with our habits, there's more to life. It is not possible to be all of our habits. These habits are our choices and can impact who we become or what we do. When we make a change to a negative habit it can change our lives. A healthy way of eating will change the way we feel about emotional eating. A happier life is a better life.

Although it may seem difficult at times to break a habit that has become so ingrained in your mind, it is possible. As humans, we know that the most comfortable habits will become our default. But once we get a new habit ingrained into our brains, there is no turning around. Once the new habit has been ingrained into our daily lives and behavior, it becomes our new source of comfort. The new habit will be just as important to us as the old one. But it will have a greater positive outcome. While we try to change our behavior, we may also be trying to live the change that we desire. There is no difference in how your brain perceives the current, more harmful habit and the new, better one. It doesn't matter what your brain recognizes as a negative or positive habit. This is why it was so important to first be aware of them. It was then possible to discern which habits we would like to continue.

It is a good idea to be aware of what habit you are trying to break. It is important to see our habits from a bird's-eye view. Take a step back from our situations and examine our habits. This will help us see the roots of our habits. You will have a better understanding about why you developed the habit. Perhaps we can have some kind of relationship to an overeating habit that began after we lose our pet dog. It's likely that emotional eating has continued even after that loss. Although we may not eat every day because we are sad, this is how our eating habits were formed. It doesn't have to be that way. Our eating habits may have formed out of no reason. It could have been that one day we discovered a passion for potato chips, and then it became a habit to indulge in potato chips every day while watching our favorite television shows. It could be as benign as regular potato consumption, or as severe as the death of our dog. It is possible to get an idea of how hard it will be for us to change our habits by finding out what the cause is. The habit that formed after losing a dog can be much harder to break than the one that started out of the blue.

You should approach the formation of new positive habits in a relationship-based manner. This is possible by telling our friends and family about the new routine. Our friends and family will often hold us accountable for the behavior and keep us motivated. This can be helpful when trying get rid of a bad habit. You can slowly decrease the negative effects of your negative behavior by replacing it with a positive one. If we can share our positive habits with other people, it will help us make the change.

Our habits have been covered extensively so far. All of this information will help us understand ourselves on an even deeper level. We now know a lot more about how habits are formed, maintained, and how to change them. This text may have allowed you to take some time to examine how emotional eating has led to these conclusions. It is probable that it began as a habit. You might have a small habit, such as frequent trips to the grocery store in the evening or more food on your plate each night. You may find that the habit can be broken depending on your circumstances. Sometimes, it may seem like so. We've got the knowledge that will keep us going. There is still hope of conquering unhealthy eating no matter how far behind you think you are. We now have all the tools we need to tackle unhealthy eating. As we continue, we will gain more ammunition. Once we have this knowledge, we can dive deeper into boring eating. It is possible to apply your personal knowledge to thoughts and emotions that are related to eating. Through it all, we can change and break the unhealthy habits that hold us back. You can do it and you are even more powerful than before. Your single realization that you want to change is enough fire under your belly. Let's break free and be like the Phoenix. It's time for our transformation--consciously changing and shifting our old ways.

Chapter 3: Happiness Effect

We are happy to think about this, right? When we think of living our best lives, it is easy to feel the fire in our hearts. We all desire to live our best lives. That's our human nature. If I were to tell you, this positive feeling plays a part in why we eat. Would you believe me? This could be because food can trigger similar feelings in us. Could that be true?! It is possible to get a positive emotional response from food. It's true. It's actually quite simple to see the science behind it and understand why we eat when we are bored. This can reveal what drives us to eat. You may be actually in pursuit of something other than eating.

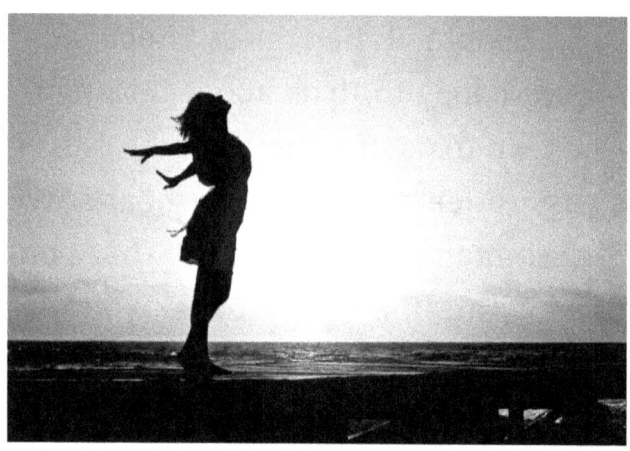

When we are thinking about positive change, it is like a flame in our souls. We can also light a spark when we visualize the things that we want. We all desire to be successful. All of these things spark some desire, regardless of whether they are a new car or a house, three children, or a beautiful home in the hills. We want to be happy and pursue these things. It's almost as if this is where we will achieve our goals. As if the journey is too hard to enjoy. We get so involved in achieving our dreams and goals that we forget to enjoy our journey. It is the journey that matters most. The thing we desire to be happy with may not bring us happiness. We should just enjoy the journey.

Similar can be said for eating. Yes, it's true. The speaker rings clear and unmistakable. People eat to find happiness. Sometimes food can bring us that feeling. One example is when we feel slightly blah. We go to the pantry for food. We take our chocolate wafers back and grab our usual snack. We enjoy our snack and feel instantly happy. We feel happy just for enjoying our little snack. But what we really are doing is telling ourselves we are bored. Then we look for a way to change our mood. The truth is that when we say we're bored, we actually feel a lack or fulfillment at the present moment. Find something that makes your heart happy. There are many things that we can do, regardless of how negative a feeling is, to get over it. There are many things we can do to relieve boredom, instead of eating. You can entertain yourself, for example, by telling yourself that you are bored in this moment. We might go for walks or play a video game. Eating isn't the only way to solve this problem.

What exactly is True Happiness?

The pursuit of happiness may seem the only way to go, but it's not. Although we can find happiness with a new car and a new home, that doesn't mean it should be pursued. Happiness does not come from a brand new car or house. It is not something we need or want to search for. It's something we can just be. It is so easy. You can be happy almost anywhere. Happiness does not come from another object, achievement or person. It is something that you can do. You can actually be happy. Even while we are driving, washing our cat, and filing taxes, it is possible to feel happy. Yes, anytime, anyplace. Happiness is something we can all achieve. Happiness doesn't have to be something you seek. It is possible to be present when we are only aware of what we are doing, and all the emotions involved. It's like the hawks' perspective, or even being aware of oneself, it allows us to see a bigger picture. It is possible to see all emotions and not be enslaved to them. It is possible to enjoy the moment and be happy, but it is important that you are aware of this first.

Instead of looking for happiness, it might be easier to accept what is. When you're fully present, it can be almost impossible to not be happy. Although there may be sadness and some grief, we see that there is still happiness. It is much easier to simply be happy. Life is happiness. We are happiness. There are so many great joys. You don't have to search for happiness or try to achieve it. Be grateful for all that you have.

There are also our feelings. We are the sum of our thoughts, emotions and feelings. Sometimes, these are things we avoid in order to find happiness. Sometimes we feel that having negative emotions could cause us to be unhappy. This is the most absurd belief. This is because the more we avoid, we cause more harm. Amazing how often we think we are doing something good when in fact it is actually causing more harm. Like when we choose to eat in order to feel better, we may be hiding the truth of how we really feel. You must face your feelings and accept them. You don't need to try and hide it, or ignore it. You may feel that your feelings aren't important or make no sense if you ignore them. No matter how strong your feelings, they are valid and important. If you are unhappy, find out why and fix it. You can feel what you want. That's all. There is no more explanation. You are simply upset. You don't need to feel miserable. Even if you are unhappy, it will pass. Happiness is the most important feeling. It's almost more than any other feeling. Enjoying the moment is the best way to allow happiness to shine through. It's all about enjoying life. It's all we have. So, feelings of sadness, anger or disgust are things that can surface and then disappear.

If we resort to eating to escape these negative emotions, we are actually doing ourself a disservice. It is making life harder for ourselves. Refusing to express your feelings can lead to negative effects on your body. Fear can be found in the lower right back. It can manifest physically. The area might feel slightly tender. If you have been there for years, it may be contributing to your physical well being, making yourself more susceptible to back aches. Not dealing with these feelings can lead to a decline in your physical health and emotional well-being. The same applies to when we replace dealing with our own emotions with eating. We can gain weight and become even more unhappy. It is not a good idea to eat to cope with these feelings. It won't solve your emotional problems in the long-term. It will just add to them later. What can you do to recognize these negative emotions? It could be fear, or any other negative emotion.

If we avoid our emotions, it can cause more problems in the future. Some people try to avoid their emotions, believing that negative feelings will make them unhappy. This is completely wrong.

Negative emotions are part of everyday life. It is normal to experience negative emotions at times. However, this does not mean we will feel unhappy. Negative feelings can be a reaction to external events. It is almost a given that we will experience feelings like sadness, anger or resentment. While they might not be positive emotions but they are worth experiencing. They are what make life worthwhile. Without the ups & downs that shape our lives, it is impossible to know what true happiness feels like. It is what makes our lives so amazing. We all experience trials, tribulations as well as difficulties and hardships. We are not limited to one emotion. We will flow and fluctuate with our emotions. It is okay to let our emotions flow. It is not healthy to not allow yourself to feel and express your emotions. You're not being true to yourself and your feelings. You can only feel what it is that you feel. There was no need for questions. You are human and you have the right of expression. Every person feels the same way as you do. Although we feel all these emotions, that doesn't mean that we are always right. We should not be confined to one feeling. Happiness must be prioritized and made a priority. This will also fluctuate. It's okay to let it happen and accept who we are. It changes constantly. However, you shouldn't cling to just one emotion and become a slave to it. You can feel your emotions and let them flow without judgment. You can cry out if you're sad. If you feel sad, you can do what makes you feel better. Keep moving on. It's not worth living in sadness every day. As with any other emotion, you shouldn't look for reasons not to be sad. Avoiding our emotions can be the most harmful.

Sometimes, it might seem scary to face your emotions. Dependent on how strong our emotions are, we may question what is wrong. Emotions are complex and frightening. It can be tempting to simply push them under the carpet and hope that they vanish. Doing this is basically telling yourself that your emotions are negative and should be judged. Instead, approach your emotions as if you are a friend offering support. Humans are defined by our emotions. If we didn't feel things, we'd just be like robots. There would be no substance in life. It would be impossible to have substance in life if we didn't embrace all of our emotions.

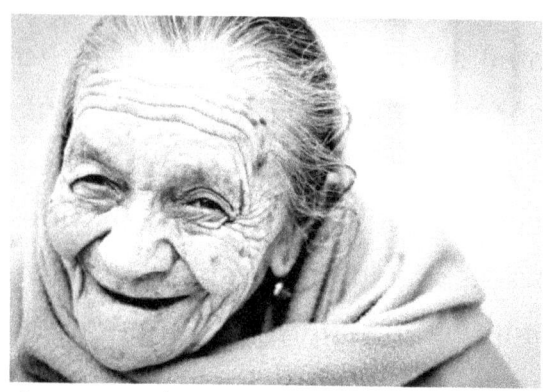

Allowing ourselves to feel emotions is a good thing. Let's say we need to be angry, and we cry. Whatever helps us cope with our feelings and relieves stress. It is wrong to pretend these feelings are harmful or that they will harm us by dealing with them. They should not be turned to food or other unhealthy coping tools to help them. We're failing to recognize emotions when we turn our attention to food. We don't recognize the emotion and avoid it. We choose to eat rather than address our emotions. If we did, we could come up with something healthier for our feelings. We can ask ourselves why we feel that way and process our emotions. You must understand your feelings and find out why. It's natural. You don't have to feel bad about your feelings. It won't make it any less natural. In fact, you might find yourself happier because you are more open to your feelings. By facing your emotions and working with them, it can help you build a healthy relationship. It allows for healthy relationships to form with others. It gives you the opportunity to express yourself and allows others to do it. You also create a space for others to express themselves and it helps build close relationships. But this doesn't mean we have to act out all the time. However, we must communicate our madness in a communicative manner. Talk about it if in doubt. Food won't help you manage your emotions or help you be productive. Food can only give you immediate relief while you ignore the monster below.

There are some signs you might be dealing in an unhealthy way with your feelings and trying to avoid them. You might notice that your boredom is often accompanied by an urge to go to the kitchen. The next time you eat food, ask yourself if you are eating it for other reasons than hunger. Are you hungry or bored? Are you angry? Any other sign than being hungry could indicate you are turning to food in order to cope with your emotions. An additional sign could be feeling anxious or depressed all the time. Sometimes these symptoms can be caused by our own thoughts. As you check in with yourself, let us return to observing what our thoughts are for a while. Do they have anything to do with our feelings? Sometimes we think feeling sad or mad is something to be critical about. It is actually quite the opposite. This is why we should not judge our feelings. I encourage you do this. To let yourself feel whatever emotions you may be feeling. When you find yourself getting upset about something, try to imagine what you would think of a friend feeling. You would most likely want to provide some relief or comfort to them. You should do it the same way to yourself. Remember that you are only human. It's normal to feel these emotions. Even if you are upset about something minor, it does not matter. Allow yourself to feel what is bothering you. While it is possible to feel sad or grievous emotions, happiness can be the most important emotion. We want to be happy. And when we feel happy others will too. We all want to have fun in our lives. It all starts with us, right here in the present moment.

Create Our Own Joy

How do we create happiness in our lives? The best thing is to use the few tools you already have. We can recognize our feelings as temporary and deal with them. It is possible to choose to feel happy anytime we like and just live the joys. It is possible to just be happy right now, for example. We can choose to be happy often if we want to live a happy and fulfilled life. Let go of your emotions and learn to observe, deal, and let them go. These life lessons are not the only ones we can learn. We can also avoid doing certain things. Although it is important to not feel unhappy, we can avoid having negative thinking that leads to unhappiness.

The important thing here is that you can choose how you feel at any time. It doesn't matter if we feel "bored", we can still choose happiness. There are always positive things to be thankful for and we can choose to see the good in every situation. Happiness is something we can choose to become. This attitude will make it easier for us to accept our negativities and allow them to pass. Because emotions are like all feelings, they fluctuate. They are fleeting. However, they can also be very positive. The key to happiness is choosing to be happy in every moment. It is possible to start by simply being happy with the little things. When we do this, it creates a domino effect on the rest of our lives. We can just be happy. It might seem farfetched, but we are only now discovering how to do it. It is possible to choose to feel happy now that we have this information.

Sometimes, we can be unhappy with ourselves and fall into destructive behaviors. It is possible to look for happiness in the wrong places. You might find yourself focusing more on the opinions of others than your own. By doing so, you may be more concerned about what others think of you than you are about yourself. You might try to please everyone but it won't make you truly happy. Because not everyone will be happy all the time. Your worth and value do not depend on what others think. It would almost be impossible to please all people you meet. It is impossible to please everyone. All you can do, is be yourself and make the changes you desire. Only do what makes your heart happy.

Second, unhappy people tend focus on the negatives more than the positives. This can be avoided if you want to feel happier. Negativity can cloud everything and creates a dark cloud. It brings down everyone and leads to lower productivity. Focusing on our own lives and striving to live the best possible life will make a huge difference in the long term. Looking at the positives will help us to be optimistic about our future. We will be more optimistic and motivated about our lives, and our health. This will make it easier to imagine the best version possible of ourselves.

Happiness and The Brain

This information can help us see how vital it is to cultivate our happiness. We all strive to be happy, but we don't realize that happiness is possible at any moment. Happiness is everywhere. Understanding the science behind happiness is key. We know we can change and create the state of our being. Our thoughts and emotions play an essential role in our well-being. However, our brain also contains certain chemicals. These chemicals are required to feel joy and happiness. These feelings are mostly caused by dopamine, serotonin, oxytocin and endorphins. Each of these produce the chemicals we need to feel good.

Let's start by talking about serotonin. While we don't yet know what chemical is responsible for our happiness and well-being, serotonin certainly plays a significant role. It is also known as the "happiness drug." It improves our feelings of well-being, confidence, and belonging. The presence of other people can boost our serotonin. Feeling valued and important by those around you can bring about this serotonin happiness. When we feel this joy, it is natural to be happy. You can get a boost in serotonin by going outside. According to some studies, sunlight can lower depression levels, improve moods, and allow for better sleeping patterns.

Dopamine, the next chemical responsible to our happiness, is also responsible. You might have heard of dopamine. Dopamine is the most important chemical in our brains and good feelings. Dopamine can be released by the brain after doing a good job, achieving a goal or having sex. Dopamine, which is released in response to these actions, is sometimes called the "reward molecules". It is important for how quickly and efficiently things can be done. It is well-known that dopamine can flood your body and reward you with feelings of happiness and fulfillment if you accomplish one of these things.

Oxytocin is third on the team responsible for ultimate happiness. This is a chemical that you might have heard of. This chemical is sometimes referred to simply as "cuddle hormone". It is the chemical your brain releases when you hug someone, cuddle or make other physical contact. It is released via the physical pathways and can also be released when we make kind gestures. This happiness hormone can be used to build closer relationships.

Endorphins will be the last happiness chemical discussed. Many of these happy feelings are much more common than we think. You may have heard the term "runners high" and wondered where it came from. You're correct! Endorphins. These are chemicals that are released in reward systems, much like dopamine. These rewarding feelings are available while you're eating, drinking or exercising. These emotions can be even released during intimate relationships. Endorphins aid the body in pain relief and increasing pleasure. They are also believed to reduce depression by exercising.

All of these happiness chemicals have great potential. We all want to feel great. You don't have to use the above-mentioned methods to activate these chemical reactions. There are other healthier options. Maybe you're single and need someone to cuddle you. You don't have to be afraid, just laughing with your loved ones can make you feel oxytocin-rich. This is a wonderful way to feel happy. It is possible to do something together such as cooking a meal. This will allow us to bond as well as share the experience of cooking a meal together. Food we love can trigger endorphins and dopamine, and we also get oxytocin from being around our loved one.

Even though eating can provide the same happiness chemicals, it's important to not allow ourselves to be influenced by its misuse. You should be able to share the many benefits of dining with your loved one, as well as spending quality time together. But eating should not be a sole enjoyment. This is something we all naturally love as humans. This is something that we should all enjoy. We should be careful about how much food we actually eat. You need to use what you've learned and be conscious of your eating habits. It's easy to overeat. But, we now realize that there are other ways to feel happy. We now know how to cope with negative feelings while still being happy. It is not possible to continue eating in an unhealthy manner. I challenge you next time you overeat, to change your behavior. Try focusing on the person instead, for example, if your friend or family member is overeating. Let's just pause and take in the moment. If you are at a restaurant, be more attentive to the conversation or scenery. You should strive for balance in your food. It doesn't matter what you eat; it also matters how you eat it. Focusing on having fun and enjoying the conversation will make us less likely to eat too much. Instead, we will be listening to each other and possibly laughing. This will help us feel happier, and not rely on food.

Food can bring joy, but it can also be dangerous. We might be in danger if food becomes a part of our daily lives. If we're not careful, we might fall prey to food addiction or obesity. We have all the tools we need to overcome these adversities and live a better, more fulfilling life. There are still temptations. It's a known fact that sugar can trigger dopamine flooding, which leads us to want to find more. Consider ants as an example. They prefer sugary crumbs to bland foods. If you eat sugary foods frequently, your brain will prefer them. It's almost impossible to resist foods such as cheesecakes, cookies, cakes, pies and cake. Sometimes it can be hard to know when to stop eating Oreos right out of the sleeves. They are both delicious and tasty. They're everywhere. It can be difficult for people to avoid these foods and choose healthier options. We know that food can be a reward and make us happy. There are many ways to be happy, even without eating. There are many other methods to increase chemical levels like dopamine. It doesn't take a lot of Oreos cookies to increase dopamine. While this may seem harmless at first, it can become very addictive. These may be the root cause of our excessive eating. Instead of looking for natural dopamine or exercises, we might just turn to food. It could be that we start eating to control our feelings. We want the exact opposite. You don't have the right to let tasty treats fools you. They're fine if you eat them for the wrong reasons.

There are many things that contribute towards our happiness, and overall well-being. You are the only one who can determine what is right. You might prefer to exercise two times a week or every other day. You might enjoy going on a long walk or taking a trip to the beach. Higher intensity activities may be better for you if you like to exercise twice weekly. It could be something like weight training, running, or even a long walk that has positive health effects. For those who are more active, it might be a good idea to choose something less strenuous.

It is best to take a walk, do yoga, or go to the gym for light exercises. These activities can help us feel more well-rounded. It doesn't matter which activity is most appealing to you. What matters is that we make every effort to be happy. It doesn't matter if you think positively or hug someone, there are many things we can do to make it possible every day. Happiness, which we all desire to be happy, is the most important thing. It is not beyond our reach, we need to remember. It is something that can be achieved by us simply being. All of the above things will make us happier. You wouldn't want to miss out on these opportunities. Happiness is something you owe to yourself. You only get one life. Don't waste a second of your time if you don't add joy to the world. Next time your car is in motion, I challenge you not to open the windows. Turn the music up.

Enjoy it however you like, whether that's listening to a podcast or driving silently. It all begins with small moments of enjoyment and, before you know, you're having fun with everything.

Chapter 4: The Future Path

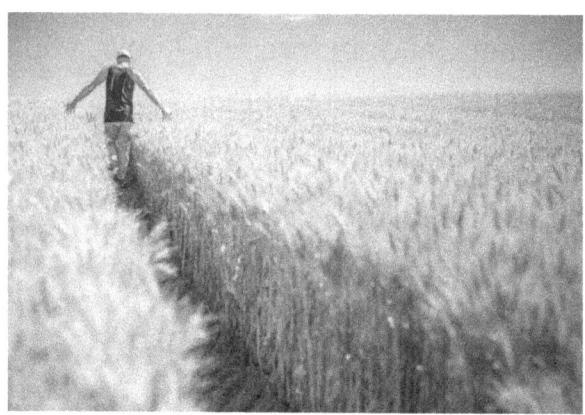

How do we get there? How can you create small moments of pleasure and ultimately enjoy everything? Since we all share similar experiences, it is no surprise that we all have them. We all have a tendency to be harder on ourself than necessary. Maybe that is what we were at first of this book. We all desire to be happy. However, we do not always see that happiness is more about a mindset than it is a destination. It is not something we find in others, material things, or our next achievement. Happiness is a way and state of being. Most happy people understand this. They also know that happiness is not found in other people or outside joys of life. It's all about them choosing to be. While we briefly discussed this, I think we all would love to know more on how we can be happy. I don't know what it is, but it could be from not eating a whole lot of Oreos.

Even though it isn't through the methods we have tried to feel happy, there are ways we can take control of our lives right now. We can make a commitment to happiness and then take action to change. Another thing we discussed earlier is one of the first things we can do. We discovered something that many unhappy people do. They are more focused on pleasing others than they are on themselves. It is possible to choose to become the best version ourselves if we wish to be happy. It's actually quite funny, if you stop to think about it. It is amazing to realize that we have the ability to be anyone we want. If we only choose to be the best version ourselves, then any phase of our lives can be the most rewarding. So, let's choose.

Our Journey:

You can start by choosing to give your all in everything you do. Let's take this example: Take the journey you are currently on. Your best effort is required at every stage. Everything from the information in this guidebook to how to implement these ideas into your daily life, you must give it everything that you have. Give it your all. If you give your best, you will find a level of satisfaction that is unmatched. Whatever the outcome, you will feel satisfied knowing you did everything you could. You will feel proud that you gave it all you had and did everything you could. You won't be able to look back at anything as you will know that you did everything you could. It was impossible to have things go differently because you gave everything your all. It is important to give it your all and not to compare ourselves to others. Doing this allows us to focus on what we want and not worry so much about what others think.

You can also choose to be happy by surrounding yourself with the right people. When we work on ourselves, it is vital that we surround ourself with people who will motivate us. People around us must inspire us. We must value them as friends and expect the same from them. Your choices about who we are around can either make or break you. When you decide to let go of people who are negative, you can live a life you love. It's too short to live in a world that makes you feel miserable. It's important that we surround ourselves not only with people who lift us up but also those who share common interests. People who are not as healthy as we are may have a greater tendency to develop unhealthy eating habits. It could impact our progress negatively if someone is not the same way. We should surround ourselves instead with people who share the same lifestyle values and goals.

Giving is another thing we can do that will bring us more happiness. Giving to others almost guarantees that we will experience the highest possible happiness. Giving can stimulate parts of the brain associated with pleasure, trust and social connection. If you give just for the sake, such as donating to a charity. You might also be releasing endorphins.

When we feel like we are helping someone, or providing service to someone else it can bring us a greater sense of fulfillment than the person receiving our assistance. It feels good to give to others. Giving to others is fulfilling, whether it's a compliment, a handout, or just a listening ear. Giving something to someone can lift your spirits if you're feeling low. While it might seem counter-intuitive, giving something to someone can actually lift your mood. Try to smile and help someone you don't know. This will lift your mood and help the stranger.

These are just a handful of ways to choose happiness. It all begins within. It's up to us to choose whether we want to help or not, who our friends are, and what we place emphasis on. It is possible to have a fulfilling and happy life. It is possible to choose happiness at any moment. You can put into practice the knowledge you have gained today. This can be done by keeping a journal of some of the things you have learned. Take a moment to appreciate what is good about your life. The future is uncertain, so the only thing we have right now is this moment. It is to be enjoyed and lived to the maximum. To do that, we must be content in the present moment.

The brain can be explored further if we take it a step further. We already know the benefits of feel-good hormones. Now we can create our own happiness. Let's now take a look at the ways that we can change our brain to feel more positive. Isn't it true that we mentioned giving as a way to make happiness. It's possible to do a kind act five times per week. Perhaps you could offer a smile to a stranger when you're on the streets. It doesn't matter how small it is, but it can make a huge difference. It's possible to hold the door open for someone, and your happiness will increase. You can teach your brain to be happier by doing this. Given that we are generally happy when we give, it makes sense that performing a kindness act will also make us happier. If you decide to do your kind act, see the effects on your mood. It's a known fact that happiness naturally increases when we do this.

The Way Forward

This may all seem daunting and difficult, but it's something that we can easily implement on our own. Moving forward requires that we remain true to ourselves. Sometimes it may feel impossible or difficult to accomplish this. Sometimes it might feel like these ideas are too difficult to put into practice in real life. I can assure that this is far from true. Sometimes we don't see how far our journey has taken. Maybe we can take the time to look at ourselves and see where we are now in order for us to start creating our happiness. You are proud of what you have accomplished for yourself. You have persevered through it all and are always eager to learn. You are learning so much, it is going to help transform you. You'll reap the rewards in the long-term. We must remember this as we transform ourselves. We can use our old self as motivation. That old version can be looked at with love, respect and let go. You don't need to dwell on all the negative aspects. We don't need to feel guilty or doubt ourselves. All that we now know, it can be easy for us to remain exactly where we are. This gives us a better view of our lives and how we eat. Moving forward, we will examine our habits and question how they were ever possible.

It can be very easy to start incorporating this knowledge, but it's important to realize how long it takes for new habits and behaviors to develop. If we recall correctly, we discovered that routine can become quite habitual. They can take on a habitual nature after some time. How long does it take for our new habits to become habitual? We are so eager to get started adding all of it to forge our new paths, so it is crucial to understand how long this will take.

Sometimes, changing habits can take longer than it seems. It can take anything from 18 days to eight months. It all depends upon the habit that we're trying to form, what our personal circumstances are, and how long it takes.

If our goal is to develop a habit such as drinking water rather than soda, it might take less for our habit to become routine. It may take longer if we want to go to the fitness center every day after work. This can motivate us to keep going even though we might want it to feel effortless right away. It doesn't matter how long it takes, so you have an open window of opportunity to work with yourself. You'll feel more free and relaxed than feeling pressured or obligated to do something. You have the freedom to move at your pace, and you shouldn't feel guilty if something happens. We should follow certain guidelines when we create our new lifestyle.

First, we must commit to the process. We have made a decision. Now it's time to commit and put in the work to form our new habits. This is where your visualization technique can help. It's easier to be committed when you have a solid reason. To take an example, if our "why", is the best version we can be, it will inspire us to be committed and determined. While it might not feel automatic or routine right away, it will get easier over time. Enjoy the process, and keep working towards your vision.

Second, be consistent. In the initial stages of developing our habitual routines, we must not lose sight of the important things. Even though we might miss a day or two down the line, it is crucial that we remain disciplined with our habits in their early stages. If we don't do this, it will make it harder for us. Your habits won't stick if you only practice them a few days per week. It is impossible to expect your habit to stick if it is only done a few days a week. Keep your habits consistent if you want them to stick. Habits that are only used occasionally can be more difficult to create. You will eventually feel so accustomed to your routine that you don't want any interruptions. It can feel almost strange or uncomfortable if you miss one day.

Third, reward your self for engaging in the habitual behavior of the day. A refreshing cup of iced coffee with your preferred creamer could be your reward. Your brain will subconsciously associate your habitual behavior with the reward. This will reinforce our existing habits. They will become more fun and something we can look forward. Understanding our bodies' needs for food is essential when creating new eating habits. It is easy to know how to make new habits, and what will work best to maintain them. But now it is necessary to know how food can affect these habits. First, different circumstances will dictate how much food we really need. A 16-year-old girl weighing in at 105lbs will have less food needs than an adult man. Your sex, health and activities, as well as your environment and any medications, will impact the recommended daily food intake. Calories help us determine how much food to consume. What our goals will also influence how much food we consume. If you are looking to lose weight, you might try to reduce your calories. This will in turn require less food. For those who want to maintain their current weight, they might need to watch what calories they consume.

Before we can create healthy eating habits, we have to first understand ourselves and the factors that affect how much food is needed. Before you can start, you need to determine your age, goals, and weight. This may seem like a common goal, but I am not sure. The first step is to figure out how many calories per day you consume. This can vary from person-to-person, as it was mentioned earlier. You should also take into account your activity level when you are calculating how many calories you will need. People who exercise a lot will need more calories than those who are more sedentary. We want to consume less calories than what we burn. You'll want to eat less calories if you're less active. However, if your activity level is higher, you will need more calories, but not more than you can eat. People who are more active might eat different foods than those who are more sedentary. You might eat more fruits or vegetables than grains. Balance is important. You can eat more one food group than another. This is something you have complete control over and can be played with. We want to be able to provide our own customized food needs.

No matter what age, there are many foods that are recommended to be eaten. No matter what diet you have, it is important that you try a variety. Whatever your needs may be, balance is the key. There are many foods you can add into your diet. Add leafy greens, such as spinach or kale, to your daily diet if vegetables are not your thing. These can be eaten as a breakfast, lunch, or dinner depending on how much they are loved. If you are not a fan, leafy greens may be added to smoothies. You can also add them to a salad, or even a breakfast sandwich for those who don't like leafy greens. Beans are another healthy food to add. Beans are a good way to get the protein we need and they're great for everyone. You can also choose beans for people who don't eat meat. People who love beans might want to add them into a taco for extra protein. They are high in fiber and are an excellent source of protein. We will end with peanut butter, which is our next food choice. Peanut butter is an irresistible food choice. Peanut butter can go with many things, such as jelly sandwiches, peanut butter and toast. You can even eat it on its own. Peanut butter is a good source of vitamins as well as antioxidants. Choose peanut butter with care. It should be free from sugar and other additives. These are just a handful of healthy food choices that we can add into our diets. It is up to each person to make the choice and experiment. The end goal is the same. Balance, moderation, & calories.

These three factors are crucial to our journey because they stop us from being too busy. It's easy to get carried away by all that delicious food. We must be mindful of our health and keep our weight under control. Overeating is a serious threat to your health. It can also cause you to lose control of your eating habits. It is more than just about how many calories you eat. Our bodies are important to us. Overeating is a bad habit that can lead to weight gain. Too much food can lead to feeling tired and sluggish. The clothes may feel tight, and you just want to lay down or take a rest. Our bodies need food to survive. This is actually how we should feel about eating. This is the first sign we should stop eating.

Overeating is not only bad for our health, but also affects our energy levels. Our digestive system works harder to digest food that we eat too often. To properly digest the food, the organs need to produce twice the amount hormones or enzymes. This can lead to stomach gas or heartburn. You will also need to make your metabolism work harder to burn all those extra calories. If this happens, you might experience heat flashes or dizziness. These aren't good for productivity and aren't healthy. We will have more trouble than we gain by overeating. Overeating does not have any benefits, except for the temporary relief we receive. This may not be worthwhile considering the many negatives.

Since we now know that eating too much may not be as beneficial in the long-term, we can conclude that it is better to only eat what we really need. Only eating what we really need allows us to live the lives we want. It is possible to feel energetic and energized so that we can get on with our day. This is how food should look. Food should fuel the mind and body. Being able to eat the right foods can help us feel happier. It is almost fun to choose healthy foods, knowing that we are making a difference in our overall well-being. While healthy foods may not look as exciting than a bag full of potato chips, there's more variety than you might think. You have so many options when it comes to the foods you can make. It is nearly never-ending. It feels thrilling when you think about it like this. Food is something that we all love. Food is something we all love as humans. Food is great, and you don't need to feel guilty after eating.

While eating healthy can be more difficult than you might think, it is definitely worth it. It's possible to experiment with endless foods and also build family bonds over your food. Even if you stick to a recipe, it's much more personal to prepare dinner with your friends and family. You can share a healthy meal, but still leave room for more. If we don't cook for our family and friends, planning ahead might be easier. For anyone who eats healthy, it is not hard to think of new ideas or cook every night. The world is busy, and it's not always easy to find the time. Planning meals ahead can help you save time. For example, you could prepare extra of your favorite recipe and have enough to last the week. So, you can use your energy for other things, and still cook a quick healthy meal. A great way to cut down on our energy is to use grains. Pasta and rice can be kept in the fridge for long periods of time. They can also be mixed with a wide variety of other foods. You can also eat beans and rice as part of your lunch or dinner. Grains can be paired with almost any meal and kept in the fridge for up to seven days. A meatless meal can be planned, so you spend less time cooking but more time eating. If we choose eggs for our protein, it will take us less time than cooking pork chops. These simple things can make our lives easier and can save us money.

All these things may sound exciting and positive. It does not necessarily mean that the transition to healthy eating will be easy. Sometimes it may be hard to stay away from our old ways. There are ways to stop ourselves from succumbing to the temptation to eat all we want. You can fill your time by planning your meals, as I have mentioned. A good tip is to drink water. Water makes us feel fuller and can be used to suppress our appetite. Water can also be used to increase calories burned, eliminate body waste and aid in workouts. Chew gum as the final way to avoid eating. Gum can, just like water can make you feel fuller. It can also reduce your cravings. Chewing gum may help you eat fewer calories, and make it easier to exercise.

We might be tempted to cave and eat anything we like, but we must remember all the good things we've done. We have taken all these steps and are ready to continue learning. Now it's time to move on and use all the knowledge we have gained into a life without emotional eating. Maybe we do still fill our boredom by eating. Now it's time to let go, and transform. This new way of life will require us live differently. If you're open to the idea of making lifestyle changes, then we can start to make them. These lifestyle changes will impact not only your physical, but also your mental health. This can be done by developing a healthy brain. The first thing we need to change in order to have a better, healthier lifestyle is our mind. Let's do it.

Chapter 5: Mindfulness Is The Key

Mindfulness will help you build a strong mind and a healthy relationship to food. The term might have been familiar to you. Mindfulness is exactly what it sounds like. Mindfulness simply means using your mind. Mindfulness refers to the ability to use your mind to be in a state that is aware. This is not only awareness but also the practice and ability to be fully present in each moment. We can practice mindfulness in relation to food. Sometimes we don't pay as much attention when eating. When we aren't paying attention, it is possible to eat more or eat less. In other words, if we don't have mindfulness, we might eat very quickly, not realizing how much food is actually being consumed.

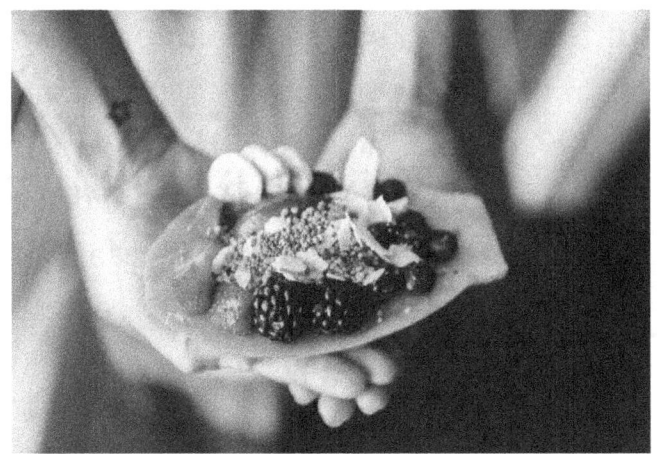

These are some of the tips and tricks we can employ to eat mindfully. It is important to eat slow and unaffected by distractions. Slow down and eat slowly when you are full. You'll notice that slowing down and eating can help you pay more attention what you eat. Doing this will allow you to pay more attention and feel the body's sensations. You'll notice when your body is full and when you should stop. When you are eating, the only thing that should be your focus is on your food. These same benefits are available when you eat without distraction. You will be able to pay more attention to your body, its sensations and emotions. This is key. This allows us to pay attention to our food, and we don't need distractions. You can, for example, watch a movie while eating. The show should not be your main concern. It is important to pay more attention to what you eat and the food you eat, than what is happening on your TV. If you can't watch TV without being distracted, then turn off the TV. This can be saved for later. However, you can still eat and look at TV without it becoming too distracting. It may be possible, provided you pay attention and pay attention to how and what you eat, as well as the physical sensations in your body.

Practicing Mindful Eating Habits

If we are able to hear our body's cues like hunger and fullness, then we need to pay attention. When we eat slower, our bodies will be more alert. It is important to eat only when we feel satisfied. The body will notify us about a quarter way through before it is full. Most likely, our body will begin to notify us when we feel full in no time. It depends on how much food you've had before, and your weight. It is common to notice the moment we are full after eating. Eat until you feel full. Be aware of your emotions and be able to judge them accordingly.

We can take our time eating mindfully and really enjoy the moment. The moment can be fully absorbed. We need to be aware of what we eat and how it tastes. It is possible to take our time and taste each flavor as we chew. It is possible to identify our favorites and those we don't like while we eat. The aroma of the food can help us prepare our bodies and minds to enjoy our meal. Take in the moment and use all our senses for enjoyment. Is your food fragrant? What does your food smell like? What smells it like? Brussels sprouts, for instance, have a more distinctive scent than other vegetables. We would avoid overeating and eating in a hurry if this were the case. Overeating causes us to eat quickly, and we often eat large quantities of food. We tend to think of 700 things when we eat in a hurry. And our attention is often diverted from enjoying our meals. Mindful eating can improve your relationship with food. Instead of focusing our attention on other things, we focus only on what's on the plate.

Also, we can be more appreciative of our food. The healthier we are with our food, the more mindful we will be. We will begin to appreciate food for its health and taste. Mindful eating can be good for us in the wider sense. Attention to small details can allow us to be more present in our bodies and less on our minds if there is a lot going on. This will allow us to pay more attention not only to the sensations within our bodies, but also to what is directly in front of and around us. A lot of times, we can lose sight on the present moment when we have many emotions to manage. Mindful eating allows us to enjoy the present moment. It will help us enjoy the moment with all its complexities.

After practicing mindful eating for a while, it will become more natural. It will not be something we have to do. At first it may feel awkward and silly. It might be difficult to accept that we need to pay attention and consider all the sensations. It is possible to try mindfulness while eating. There are many distractions that can distract you from eating out. There are many distractions, but none that can distract us from the food we are eating. Similar to the TV example above, we can be focused on our surroundings and the conversations around us while still making sure that our eating is the most important thing. Our main topic can still be our food.

When we eat, we can notice the processes taking place. That is, we can be aware that what we're doing is actually happening. It is a bodily function. It all begins with the act of eating. Our focus should be on chewing as we inhale our food. This is the first part of eating. This is the first step in chewing. Instead of chewing food at lightning speed, slow down. This could lead to slow eating. Our food should be chewed thoroughly and savored every bit. There is a purpose behind chewing food. You don't just need to eat it all. Mastication refers to chewing. This process breaks down large food particles into smaller ones. It takes two seconds to chew. If this happens, the mastication process is not properly functioning. In turn, our digestive systems work twice as hard for large food particles to be broken down. Our chewing actually moistens, and even dissolves, food during the mastication stage. For this to happen correctly, it is essential that you chew your food thoroughly. It is possible to chew slowly and allow food to flow smoothly. This allows us to taste the food. This will make eating more enjoyable if it is done right. It is possible to taste the food and also feel it change in texture when we chew slowly. If we pay more attention, we can actually feel our food dissolve. This will improve our experience of eating, and it will engulf you in the moment. You will be able eat less food, but still have the satisfaction of eating. To become more mindful of the food that we are eating, it is possible to chew slowly and in smaller quantities. It will be much more enjoyable than eating small pieces of food quickly without tasting.

A second way to practice mindful eating is to eat only when you feel hungry. When we are more familiar with mindful eating, our bodies will be more alert to our cues. Instead of eating to soothe our emotions, we'll eat just for the sake. We can remember the quote from earlier in the book.

"Eat to nourish your body, not just your emotions."

It is important to remember this quote. Listening to our body's cues will help us recognize them. We can tune in to our body and eat when it is hungry. Instead of eating to satisfy our emotional needs, we will eat in order to satisfy the hunger pangs. We will eat only to satisfy our appetites and fuel our bodies.

We shouldn't delay eating until we feel absolutely starving. Doing this will make us eat more than what we really should. Also, we are causing more harm than good to our bodies. Some may believe that by being hungry we help ourselves lose weight. This isn't true. Our bodies store fat when we feel starving. This means that we will burn fewer calories if we don't eat enough. In essence, you are giving your body an idea that it must conserve its resources in order to get what it needs. It is okay to not eat until you feel full, but it is also important to eat only when you are feeling hungry. You don't get any benefit from starving yourself.

This can lead us astray to believe that smaller portions are better. This is actually true. In fact, eating smaller meals more often can do the opposite to what starving will. Our blood sugar will plummet if we are starving ourselves. This can lead to a craving for sweeter foods. Our blood sugar levels will be more stable if we eat in smaller portions. You can also eat smaller meals to satisfy your appetite, rather than ignore it. It provides nutrients to your body instead of depriving yourself of them. In fact, smaller meals more often can actually help to increase your metabolism. This can help with weight loss. But, starving yourself will slow down our metabolism. When we are well-nourished, our metabolism works better and can use fats, carbohydrates, protein, and fats to fuel our bodies. If we do not satiate our hunger and skip meals we make our body store fat rather then use it. To have energy and fuel throughout our day, our bodies require nutrients from food.

Mindful eating offers many benefits

It all boils down to being mindful. All that is required is to pay attention to what we eat. All that is important is to focus on our food. It is important to eat slowly, focus on what you are eating, avoid distractions, and eat until you feel full. This tool will help us get back control of our bad eating habits. It will make food more pleasant and will help us feel balanced and clearer. It will make it easier to eat healthy, as well as allowing us to pay more attention and fully enjoy our food. This will bring us more joy than filling a void. We might start to see positive effects when we learn to eat mindfully. It can give us a whole new level in awareness that we didn't have before.

Mindful eating can also be helpful in reducing binging. Being mindful of our food and slowing down will help us to eat less. Binge eating can make us forget about the physical sensations that our body is experiencing. Our bodies don't know what is happening. We may eat out of boredom or because we are bored. When we become more aware and conscious of the sensations in our bodies, we can begin to identify when we are feeling full. Instead of eating until you feel sick or uncomfortable, eat until you feel satisfied. Emotional eating, another issue mindfulness can reduce, is also reduced. Emotional eating can be reduced by mindfulness. We will not be focusing on our food or the sensations of our bodies. It won't be about eating to satisfy our emotions, but mindful eating.

As you can see mindful eating can help with a variety of things. You can feel joy and peace, overall. You can be mindful when you eat and also when you shop for food. In a previous article, we discussed the benefits of eating healthy foods as opposed to the pleasure from eating a bag of Oreos. Oreos may be a treat that we enjoy occasionally, but it's important to remember to buy groceries with care. Oreo cookies are not healthy, so we shouldn't go out to buy them. Here are some steps you can follow the next time that you go to the grocery shop.

First of all, choosing the right foods to eat is an easy decision. By this I mean that we have the choice to eat only natural food. Oreos don't fall within this category. Real foods will be found in the produce section. There are also authentic and raw meats nearby. This will prevent you from having to buy many cookies and allow you to enjoy your meals. This saves you time later. Even though the meat and produce section is not the only place where you can find real food, it's important to pay close attention to nutrition labels. If some ingredients are nearly impossible to pronounce, it is best to avoid adding them to the shopping cart. These foods contain unknown ingredients that are difficult to identify. These foods are likely to be nearly as unhealthy as processed foods. These are dangerous and we should avoid them as much as possible. These are more harmful than Oreos for our health, so we should avoid both.

It is possible that we are not the only person shopping for food. This can cause problems. Others in your household may not be following the same healthy lifestyles as you. Oreos and other treats for small children might be required. If this is the case, it's important to get your entire family on the same page. They should have a clear idea of what you can eat and what you should avoid. Once they have this information, it should be possible to agree on a compromise. It might be possible to keep junk food at a safe place, or to purchase as little as possible. Your family should be able to understand your feelings and show respect.

You can also be mindful while shopping or eating. A food diary can help you to keep track of your meals. A food diary records the information you eat, drink, and when. This allows us to keep track on our food intake and calories. Keep a daily log of all your food and drink intake to ensure a complete food diary. We might not know what we ate at any given moment. Being mindful can help us be more aware of what foods we eat. To make it easier to change our eating habits, keep a food diary each day. You might notice that you should be eating less of one food type than the others. It is possible that we have eaten too much meat over the course of the week. You can substitute more vegetables for meat and reduce the amount you eat. It can be helpful to keep track of the reasons we eat. It is possible to track which foods we eat according to how we feel. You can start to change your eating habits by noticing when you eat unhealthy foods.

Also, a food journal can help you plan your meals more efficiently. You can be more detailed about the details when planning your meals with a food journal. One example is to write down the time we will eat each meal. This allows us to plan ahead and visualize the times we will eat. This can help us eat breakfast more often or get dinner ready earlier.

You can put your focus on the food and think of what you could cook that would fit into your schedule. Perhaps we'll make overnight oatmeal if we don't have much time in the mornings. It's easy to grab and go but still have a healthy meal. It is important to keep track when changing things like this. You might miss a dinner or eat less than you planned. This is something that we need to keep track of, especially if we want to adopt healthy eating habits.

It is possible to improve your eating habits by slowing down, becoming more mindful and becoming more present. Mindfulness is something that can be practiced by eating. We have already mentioned that we can find our greatest happiness by simply enjoying the moment. A great example of how mindfulness can affect other areas is slowing down, and becoming completely immersed into our meals. You can choose to feel like this at any time. You can practice mindfulness the next time that you drive your car. Be aware of all that you see. You can take the time to observe what it feels like to be sitting in that seat. Take note of what you see as you drive. Pay attention and pay attention to the sounds all around you. These sounds will help you become more aware of the present moment. They will also make you feel happy. It is possible to feel joy when you are completely present in the moment. It's as easy to be present and mindful. As you can see, eating can be a fun and enjoyable experience if we are more conscious of it.

Mindful eating is a great way to eat mindfully. You have to weigh the pros and con's before you can start. Some adjustments may be required in our lifestyles, and we might need to have patience. All in all, though, it is well worth it. Why wouldn't we want to enjoy every bite? It's also completely healthy. How could that be possible? Aren't healthy things less enjoyable? The practice of mindfulness only enhances the enjoyment of something everyone already enjoys. Imagine how amazing life would be, if we lived every moment mindfully. Mindful eating, however, is possible. This will only require some adjustments at the beginning.

All in all mindfulness is the key to most things. It will help us overcome our bad eating habits and lead a happier, more fulfilling life. Mindfulness will take you to the vision you have of your best self. Nothing can bring you more satisfaction than seeing the finish line and feeling that you've been fully present every moment. This is how you achieve your greatest happiness. It will make us feel happy when we look back on our lives. This mindfulness can also be transferred to other areas, which will make them all the more worthwhile. This will be made possible by being more mindful about our workouts and bodies. A part of your goal to lose weight is to feel happy. When we look at ourselves now, our eating habits can cause us to feel miserable. You can create the body image and lifestyle you want. This will increase your self-esteem, confidence in all aspects of your life, and drive. This will help you feel transformed if you're mindful. You will feel a shift. While you might not be able to walk out with six-pack abs from one session of gym, you can feel the difference. You can make this exercise as enjoyable as eating. It's worth being mindful of the sweat on your skin, as you work to become your best. You can simply be aware of everything and feel the positive effects of your progress.

Mindful eating will be our salvation when it comes down to creating healthier eating habits. Mindfulness will make us more aware of how we eat. This is how we can identify when we eat out of boredom and if we really are hungry. Mindfulness can help us change our perception that we are bored. Realizing how happy we can simply be in the present moment makes it seem silly to claim we are bored. There's so many things happening at the moment that we can't be bored. Even if this is true, it's important to find other ways of entertaining boredom. Eating is not the answer. Doing so means that we do not pay attention to what we are eating. This is a negative emotion that we choose to resolve by eating. This is not the reason for eating. It takes away the joy of eating.

We can develop a healthy relationship between food and our emotions by practicing mindfulness.

Chapter 6: What Is Binge Eating Disorder And How Can It Be Treated?

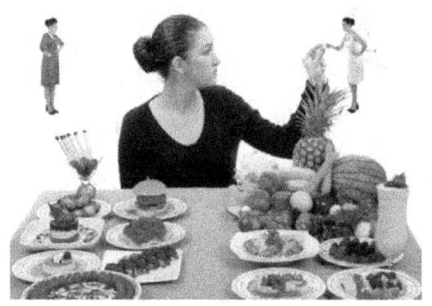

Binge refers to excessive eating. Binge can be described as excessive indulgence.

Binge Eating Disorder (BED) is a serious disorder that can cause recurring episodes. This disorder causes at most two episodes per week. They feel powerless to stop them from having it happen. Due to the feelings of helplessness and despair they felt while binging, many feel extreme anxiety.

Many people suffering from stress often find themselves in a vicious cycle. In order to feel better, many sufferers resort to binging when under stress. However, binging can make them feel worse than before. As they get the immediate pleasure from large amounts of food, many people keep doing it again and again. They feel depressed afterward, which leads to a cycle where they eat more food until they feel better. It's a vicious cycle that can be difficult to break. However, there are ways you can get it broken with some hard work. Once an individual decides that they want to seek treatment and becomes determined to make positive lifestyle changes, the change will begin.

Eating Disorders: Many eating disorders can be described as psychiatric diseases that alter normal eating patterns. These disturbances can result in significantly impaired psychosocial function and physical health. American Psychiatric Association, (APA) has identified the diagnostic criteria for the most prevalent eating disorders. These include Anorexia Nervosa Bulimia Nervosa Bulimia Nervosa Bulinge Eating Disorder, Bulimia Nervosa and Binge Eating Disorder. These disorders cause serious eating problems, such as binging or restricting your intake. These conditions can lead to serious concerns about the body's appearance and weight. Common eating disorders can affect adolescents both as girls and young women. However, 40 percent of cases in binge eating disorder and 5% - 15% in cases of anorexia nervesa are experienced by teenage girls. Eating disorders are more common than in industrialized countries and can be found in all major ethnicities and socioeconomic levels. These eating disorders can be caused by a combination of neurochemical and developmental genetic, sociocultural and sociocultural factors.

Bulimia-nervosa refers to a condition that involves regular binge eating and is followed by a strategy that will prevent weight gain. These can include self-induced vomit, diuretic misuse, laxative misuse, fasting, and compulsive exercise. The compensatory behavior of binge-eating and compulsive exercise are often seen at least two times per week for three to four months.

Anorexianervosa refers to self-starvation. This can eventually lead to emaciation. Anorexic patients often fear becoming obese or gain weight. These concerns can be expressed even though they have no weight. These concerns often lead to people starving themselves to the point of death or life threatening.

Binge eating disorder is similar in nature to bulimia. However there is no attempt to cleanse the food. Most people with binge eating disorder are obese. People who are affected by it may also be suffering from night eating disorder (NES). This is a condition that occurs when most of the daily energy intake happens after dinner.

The Characteristics of Binge Eating

Feeling or Sense Of Pleasure. The first few moments of binging are filled by pleasure. The pleasant sensation of eating the food is due to the way it smells, tastes, and textures. These feelings of joy usually last only a short time. These feelings of pleasure will soon be replaced by feelings of disgust or repulsion as they consume more food.

Binge-eaters can feel ashamed of their actions and feelings of repulsion. However, they will continue to eat.

Fast/Rapid Eating. These people tend to eat quickly when they are having a binge. They eat fast because they don't want to slow down and think about the bad eating habits they have. Binge-eaters often stuff their faces with food, and don't take the time to chew.

Cravings and feelings of desperation to eat. A binge eating disorder that many binge-eaters find embarrassing and degrading is the need to eat. Not all binge eaters experience these feelings. However, some feel they can't stop eating because of these intense cravings. Some binge-eaters resort to shoplifting or stealing food items, while others eat food they have stolen.

Zombie-like Trance. Some binge-eaters described feeling as if they were in a zombie trance, while their binges were on. It was like having no control, or being on autopilot while binging. They may also continue to read or watch television while binging. This is to stop them worrying about what else they might be doing.

Loss of self-control Binge-eating causes people to feel like they don't have enough self-control to stop eating. When they eat, they cannot stop it from happening again. The feeling of helplessness that occurs when they realize they have eaten too many calories, but still continue to eat.

It is best to keep it a secret. The most common characteristic of bingeing is the inability to keep it a secret. Binge-eaters are ashamed of their eating habits, so they hide them as much as possible. Binge eaters will indulge in their binging habits alone. They will eat normally when they're with others to hide their disorder.

(Table of Contents).

Chapter 7: What Signs And Symptoms Are Possible In Binge Eating

If you find yourself constantly thinking about food, or if your eating habits make you feel sick, then you may have an eating problem. These are the clear signs and symptoms for binge eating disorder. Are you secretly eating, ashamed to eat after eating, and unable to stop? Do you use food as a way to get away from stress and anxiety? These are just two of the many questions you should be asking.

Signs. Binge-eating can lead to obesity, but others may appear normal. It can be hard to tell if someone is suffering from compulsive, or emotional eating. It is possible to recognize binge eating disorder by observing certain behavioral and emotional signs.

Symptoms. Binge-eating disorders can still be treated. They often binge eat when they are alone. They are often unable to set a time and they eat at any hour. They feel ashamed of their eating habits, and they are embarrassed at how much they eat. This is why they eat in secret. They keep food stocks for later consumption. They may not be able, even though they are full, to stop eating excessive quantities of food. Most people binge eat at nights. After a long day at the office, most people will go home to indulge in their food.

Many binge-eaters believe they can only relieve stress by binging. They have come to associate food with happiness and love, and they are happy. They will never be satisfied no matter how much food they consume. This can lead to depression and a negative outlook on their eating habits. As they look for comfort, their feelings of depression can lead them to overeat.

Later, binge-eaters seek ways to manage their weight and improve their eating habits. They will then attempt to reduce their food intake while trying to eat normal, balanced meals. It ends up that their stress over a restricted diet leads them to eat more and to re-invent themselves while trying to manage the stress.

Many people suffering from this disorder have erratic weight loss and weight gains, which can be described as a yo/yo effect. Some are having trouble losing weight. Although binge-eating disorder can be extremely difficult to treat, there is an easy solution. If you suspect that your loved one has the disorder, it's best to have an open and honest conversation with them and get professional help from a doctor or nutritionist. To be successful with treatment, you must have self-determination. If someone needs treatment, they need to be willing to receive help and will have to go through it in order to succeed in reducing their emotional eating.

(Table of Contents).

Chapter 8: The Complications Binge-Eating People Can Expect

Binge eating disorder can affect anyone. The condition typically begins in late adolescence, or early adulthood. This condition is 1.5 times more common among women than in men. There are several factors that may increase the risk of someone developing it. This disorder can be caused by both risk factors or causes.

Causes. Binge eating disorder can often be viewed as a person's attempt to overcome low self-worth, unhappy life, and lack of satisfaction. This disorder can have many cultural, biological, social, psychological, or psychological causes. Research has shown that certain genetic mutations may lead to an addiction. The hypothalamus, which is dysfunctional, could be another cause of binge eating disorder. Hypothalamus dysfunction is another form of abnormality that could lead to binge eating disorder. It is an endocrine organ that controls appetite. Hypothalamus dysfunction can lead to inaccurate information about hunger and satiety.

Research has shown that serotonin (a brain chemical) can influence a person's eating behavior. Deficiency in serotonin could lead to cravings for sweets, and other carbohydrate-rich foods like chips. Some hormones are more active in binge-eaters than in those who aren't.

Psychological problems are the main reason for binging. People with low self-esteem and confidence are more susceptible to developing it. They are often unable to express their feelings and turn to food for comfort. Although they feel relief from their fears and stress, overeating makes them feel isolated. They may feel better for a short time when they eat. They will quickly feel upset when they realize the amount they have eaten. Binge eating can also be triggered by past traumas. An individual who is unhappy with how they look, or lacks self-confidence, will be more susceptible to this condition.

Culture and society can influence how an individual eats. People can also be more likely to develop an eating disorder when they feel pressured by society to achieve a certain type of body image. A person's shame about their appearance can lead him or her to become more self-conscious, which eventually leads to an increase in weight. It is also more likely that people who were overweight as children are at higher risk for developing this disorder. These disorders can be linked to parents who reward their children with food.

Binge eating can lead to other health problems. These may be social, psychological, emotional or physical in nature. It can lead to depression, anxiety, substance abuse, and possibly even suicide if not treated immediately.

Binge eating can have the most severe physical consequences, such as weight gain that could lead to obesity. Obesity can lead to cardiovascular diseases such as elevated blood pressure and high cholesterol. It could also lead to osteoarthritis, cancer, and diabetes. Other conditions that could be present include gastrointestinal problems as well as joint pain, muscle pain and gallbladder disease. Women may also experience menstrual issues. These complications could be life-threatening and should not be ignored.

A lot of foods people choose to binge eat are often low in nutrients and high in fats and sugar. Cookies, chocolates and jams are just a few examples. These foods are known to cause serious health problems. The binge-eating behavior of binge eaters can lead to other complications.

(Table of Contents).

Chapter 9: What Psychotherapy Treatments, & Medications Would Work?

Mental illnesses can include Binge Eating Disorders. Most of these disorders do not respond to medication. If untreated, these disorders can cause irreversible and degenerative brain and nervous system tissue damage. These are not only behavioral issues. To address the underlying cause, these conditions will require medical, nutritional, and often pharmacological treatment.

Binge eating disorder can be treated just like any other eating disorder. Strategies include dietary management and nutrition counseling, as well group and one-on-one psychotherapy, and medication. Some treatment programs will be primarily focused on weight-loss, nutrition counseling, and other areas. It has been shown that this treatment alone can reduce binge eating episodes and prevent weight-loss regressions.

There are also programs that target binge eating episodes and not weight-loss. Treatment for someone who binges is to improve self-acceptance, body image, physical activity, nutrition, and overall health.

Psychotherapy. Studies have shown that the use of psychological therapy alone is effective in treating binge eating disorders. These studies are based on the fact that therapy teaches many lessons to the patients. These include learning how to deal with binge eating and managing their stress.

Psychotherapy is a key component of a comprehensive treatment of binge eating disorders. However, many people who have it need other therapies. This is because binge eating disorder is more than just a psychological problem. It is also an issue of nutrition.

These are the treatments available to those with binge eating disorders.

Dialectical Behaviour Therapy (DBT) DBT therapy focuses on both emotional and behavioral issues. These treatment methods help binge-eaters to learn how to control their emotions, handle stress better, overcome conflicts, and be more accepting of themselves. This therapy will also challenge unhealthy attitudes and beliefs patients may have about their body, diet, or food choices. It teaches patients to accept difficult emotions and move forward.

DBT is available on a weekly basis for both individual and group therapy. It is based around four modules of therapy: interpersonal effectiveness (emotion regulation), mindfulness (mindfulness), and distress tolerance.

Interpersonal Psychotherapy is (IPT). This type of therapy focuses primarily on patient's relationship problems and how they have affected their eating habits. It examines how binge-eating disorder sufferers relate to other people and how those relationships may contribute to their inability control over their eating habits. The therapists focus on helping patients improve their communication skills in order to have better relationships with their loved one. The emotional support that the family and friends provide will improve as the patient's communication skills improve. This support system helps patients resist the urge to binge.

Cognitive Behavioral therapy (CBT). CBT is considered the gold standard in binge eating treatment. CBT therapy focuses on helping patients recognize their illogical thoughts, and using several interventions to help them make positive changes in their thinking processes. This therapy helps patients recognize the triggers that cause binging episodes. These patients are taught how to avoid situations like these and how they can cope with stress without eating. CBT helps patients learn to understand their dysfunctional behavior and how to change their thoughts and feelings about weight, diet, and body images.

Medications. There are no medications that can treat binge eating disorder. But, medications can have a significant effect when used with other treatment programs, such psychotherapy, support groups and self-help techniques.

Below is a list of two medications that can be used to treat binge-eating disorders.

Anticonvulsant. Topiramate (also known as Topamax) is a seizure drug. It is also used to reduce patients' desire to binge eat. The drug helps reduce weight by decreasing patient's appetite. Topamax, like many drugs, can also cause side effects such as fatigue, dizziness, tingling in the hands, dizziness, and a loss of concentration. Inability to sweat could also result in heatstroke or glaucoma. Topamax patients who are on the medication must be in close contact with their medical providers, especially if they have severe side effects.

Antidepressants. A few studies have shown that antidepressants can be used to keep binging episodes under control.

A number of studies have shown that people who take antidepressants to control their emotions can greatly reduce the frequency of binging. Antidepressants can be used to reduce anxiety, depression, or guilt. These are all factors which can lead to binging. Antidepressants can help reduce binge-eating if they are taken for a long time.

They can regulate neurotransmitters within the brain that are responsible to controlling hunger, satiety or mood. For those with binge eating disorders, it is important to continue taking antidepressants. This will prevent a relapse from happening.

Tricyclic antidepressants and selective serotonin reuptake inhibits (SSRIs), are the most widely used antidepressants.

TCAs. These medications improve mood and relieve depression. They hinder the absorption norepinephrine and serotonin, which makes them more readily available for brain use. TCAs can be purchased in most drugstores. Norpramin is, Tofranil, Vivactil and Tofranil are all available. Side effects can occur, such as blurred vision or increased appetite, constipation, increased sweating, stomach upset, and drowsiness. These medications are typically given in very low doses to start with, and then gradually increased to reduce the risk of side effects.

You should not self-prescribe antidepressants. They could prove deadly. Before you start taking any medications, it is important to consult a qualified health professional.

SSRIs. These medications are thought to increase brain serotonin, which leads to improved mood and eating habits. Luvox is the most widely used SSRI, while Prozac is another. Side effects are possible with SSRIs. They are generally less bothersome than the TCA side effects. Side effects that are most commonly associated with SSRIs include loss of appetite, constipation or diarrhea, dizziness, low sex drive, nausea and insomnia. These side effects will likely diminish with time and be less common.

Chapter 10: A Healthy Regimen With A Good Support Group

Binge eating disorder can be almost as bad as a food addiction. It is hard to treat. The person suffering from this condition must change their eating habits to avoid relapse. If you are suffering from excess weight because of eating unhealthy food, it is time to start a reducing program. You can lose weight safely and effectively with a reducing lifestyle.

It is easy to lose weight. It takes determination and patience to achieve lasting weight loss. It is essential to be able to persevere with healthy diets. The results of a healthy weight-reduction diet take time. You can lose weight by following a diet that reduces calories. The body will not crave food as it is not starved.

Short-term weight loss can only lead to a person feeling unhappy, dissatisfied and cranky. It will be difficult for someone suffering from binge eating to succeed on a short-term diet.

Effective weight loss programs can be more successful when they are combined with support groups and therapy. It is a really good idea to have a professional nutritionist-dietitian help to arrange a meal plan that will be balanced and have the nutritional requirements that are needed by supervising the regimen.

Start a Healthy Lifestyle. You must have patience and perseverance to reach your long-term goal of a healthy weight. You don't have to lose weight to achieve your ideal body weight. Smart choices are essential to achieve your ideal weight. To be successful in losing weight, you must recognize that it takes effort.

Permanent Lifestyle Improvements It is crucial to know that temporary weight-loss cannot be achieved by following a diet. These will produce short-term results. It is essential that a person makes changes to their food choices and gets rid of unhealthy eating habits in order to reach the desired weight. To help someone suffering from bingeing, adding exercise to your lifestyle is a great way to overcome the condition and ultimately maintain a healthy weight.

Get support. A support system is a great help for those who struggle with serious conditions like binge eating. This support can be provided by a friend, family member, or even a close friend. They will find it extremely helpful to have a support group that will keep them focused and motivate them to achieve their goal of a healthier lifestyle.

You must be patient. One to two pounds per week is the goal for a good diet. Individuals who lose large amounts of weight quickly will feel tired and weak. This is unhealthy and can have detrimental effects on the mind and body. Do not rush to lose weight. It is not the fat that will be lost, but precious water and muscle.

S.M.A.R.T. weight-loss goals. Plan your weight loss plan. To keep yourself on track, you need objectives. S.M.A.R.T targets are specific, measurable. They must be achievable and realistic. They also have a time limit. In order to lose weight, the goal must contain the target weight along with the date of achievement. It is important to be realistic in setting these targets and to make them achievable.

The right tools for monitoring and evaluating your progress are essential. For you to be able to evaluate your progress, it is important that you have a monitoring system and an evaluation system. Once you have all the tools, you can assess whether your program is working. If the tools aren't sufficient, you can make the program work better by adding more. It will be easier to track your progress if you have the basic tools like a food journal, weighing scale, or measuring tape. These assessments need to be conducted on an ongoing basis. It is easier to lose weight if you are more aware and focused on your efforts.

Tips for Healthy Dieting. Avoid Fad diets also known "pitfall" diets. These diets are short-term weight loss plans that are not meant to succeed. Unfortunately, many people fall for these types of diets. These people are often overweight and are desperate to lose weight. They try many weight-loss programs without doing much research. Make sure you do your research before you begin any diet plan.

Fad diets are dangerous and unrealistic. They make the person feel deprived because they cut out a whole food group, such as carbs or fats. A proper weight loss diet will contain balanced foods and a wide range of foods. Fad diets may seem effective in the beginning. You will have to eliminate certain foods from your diet in order for you to reduce your overall calorie intake. It will only increase your desire for more food once the weight loss program is complete. The result is a new weight gain, and possible serious health problems.

Short-term diets can offer high-end products such as prepared meals or premium shakes and juices. These diets are extremely expensive and difficult to maintain long term. A lot of these special products can lead often to nutritional deficiencies. It is important to be aware of any advertisements for weight-loss product. Many are simply not realistic.

It is time to stop emotional eating. Binge-eating disorder sufferers will look for comfort in food. It is important for people with binge eating disorder to recognize and understand the triggers that cause them to eat excessive amounts of food. While there are several ways to end emotional eating, it may take some time. Try to help someone you know who is feeling stressed out and turning to food to calm down, to get them to think about other options. Perhaps they could consider doing some exercise to relieve stress.

You might find relaxation exercises like yoga, meditation, and massage helpful. A nap may be a good option if they are feeling tired and lacking in energy. This could play a role in stopping them from emotionally eating. If they're in a position where they cannot take a nap, they need to find other ways to distract them. A good way to distract yourself is to listen and watch upbeat music.

Reaching out is the best thing for those who are feeling bored or lonely. It will help them be happier if they have someone to chat and laugh with. You could take the person out in public with very limited funds to avoid temptation to buy junk food.

You can practice mindful eating. Mindful eating involves paying attention to what you eat and focusing only on the eating experience. It doesn't allow eating while you do other activities like reading, watching TV or working. Mindless eating refers to eating when you are not actively engaged in other activities. This can often lead us to eating too much without even realizing. Mindful eating means that one must focus fully on what they eat to prevent overeating. By doing this, one will be more aware of how much food they eat. This is a useful strategy that people who are binge eaters can adopt.

Mindful eating means that a person will try to experience the texture, smell, taste and textures of the foods they eat. Slowly eating and chewing the food is a good way to do this. It is almost like eating a food evaluation. Your experience with food will be enhanced if you chew them longer. Chopsticks may be a good option to help you concentrate on eating.

Your food environment is important. Your food environment can include the foods you eat, your eating habits, food preferences, and the process of food preparation. It is all about the person's eating habits. How someone takes care of their eating environment will affect their success or failure with weight-loss.

Research has shown that eating large portions of the daily recommended calories for breakfast can lead to weight loss. The metabolism can be boosted by eating a healthy and substantial breakfast. It can make a person feel satisfied and not hungry all the time. It can lead to prolonged disinterest in food and more time for the body to burn calories from breakfast. It's also a good idea if meals and snacks are planned in advance. It is not just about setting a time to consume them, but also ensuring that the quantity of the meal is planned.

A schedule can stop someone from overeating during non-scheduled hours.

To lose weight, eat less food. Instead of eating food straight from the packages, use smaller containers and plates. It will make portions appear bigger by using smaller containers. It is easier to keep track of what was eaten and how much.

Foods that are easy to access and easily available will affect your diet. It is important that you choose the right food for your health. Remember that snack foods and prepackaged food are often high-calorie, particularly in sodium and fats. They are not healthy food. Making your own meals is the best way to eat healthy foods. You'll have complete control over what ingredients you use and how much of each meal you eat.

You should always have a shopping list ready before you go. It will be easier to stay on track if you have a well-thought out list. Avoid high-calorie snacks.

Enjoy your favorite foods. Make sure to not overeat. Learn how to enjoy your favorite foods and not overeat when trying to lose weight. It doesn't matter if your weight-loss journey is healthy. You are allowed to indulge in high-calorie snacks, such as ice cream. You'll just be more inclined to crave them if these items are removed from your diet.

It is better to eat these foods less often and in smaller amounts. You can mix high-calorie snacks and healthy foods. You might want to combine ice-cream and berries. This will make your snack much healthier. This will make you feel less restrictive about your diet.

You might even consider adding indulgence to your life. It's possible to have a small bite of brownie every day for lunch, or a slice of thin marble cake on Sunday. Indulgences can be incorporated into your routine to reduce cravings for them. It is better to make sweet snacks yourself. You can lower the amount of sugar used in them. Stevia, a sugar substitute, can also be used in recipes.

High fiber foods can be a healthier choice. You'll feel more satisfied if you include fiber rich foods into your diet. Fiber-rich foods take longer to digest because they are more bulky. Fiber-rich foods give people the feeling of being satisfied right away. High fiber foods include whole grains, fruits, vegetables, legumes, and whole grains. The fiber in fruits and vegetables is not only high, but so are their water contents. You may feel fuller for longer than you are consuming calories. It is for this reason that fiber-rich food is an essential part of weight reduction diets. These foods are rich in vitamins and minerals. It is easy to include these foods in any meal.

You can enjoy fruits as snacks or desserts. Or, you can add them to high-fiber breakfast cereals. Vegetables come in many forms: raw, cooked, as main dishes, or as ingredients in salads. You can enjoy legumes as an individual or in salads or main meals.

Healthy living is possible. It can take some time and effort. When you achieve a healthy lifestyle, all of your hard work and determination will be worthwhile. Even if your exercise time is minimal, adding some exercise to your daily routine is a good idea. Drinking plenty of water throughout your day is also important. Water intake can give you the feeling of fullness and many other health benefits. Avoid sugar-laden drinks like sodas and fruity juices.

Weight-loss can be prevented by getting a good night of sleep every night. Ghrelin, and leptin are the hormones that stimulate appetite. Studies have shown this. Leptin informs the mind about hunger and satiation. A person suffering from sleep deprivation will experience an increase in ghrelin while their levels of leptin drop. This can lead to obesity and weight gain.

It is therefore important to get eight hours of sleep every night. It is actually more efficient to sleep than to watch TV or engage in other sedentary activities. Regular visits with your healthcare provider are an integral part of a healthy lifestyle. Also, it is important not to misuse drugs or drink alcohol. Tobacco use is also an undesirable habit and should be stopped as it can lead you to lung cancer.

Your support team. It can be difficult to change binge eating habits if you have been suffering from it for a long period of time. Many people avoid talking about their binging issues for years, as they find it easier to hide the episodes from their loved one. There are setbacks that can occur even with multiple treatment options. It is vital that the person suffering binge eating disorder has support and encouragement from family and friends. They also need to be monitored and receive supportive advice from their healthcare providers. People with binge eating disorders may decide to either join a formal therapy group, self-help support groups or both.

Support Groups In support groups, participants lead their own discussions.

Facilitators rotate between them from time-to-time. A trained professional may guide or lead them. The participants are able to support each other because they have had or are currently going through the same bad experiences. They can offer advice and encouragement to one another.

Chapter 11: The Self-Management Strategies That Will Help You Take Control

Bingeing disorder is not something you can treat yourself. It will be beneficial to receive some reinforcement from the treatment programs as well as some self-management strategies. These are important if you want to end binge-eating permanently. Without effective strategies, it is very difficult to achieve a healthy lifestyle.

Avoid unhealthy dieting. If people are restricted or depriving themselves of food, they will end up craving more. It is much better to know and implement effective weight management strategies instead of going on unhealthy diets.

Find nutritious foods that you like and enjoy eating them. Make sure you eat only enough to satisfy your appetite and not too much. You should make conscious and careful choices when dieting. These are safer and easier ways to lose weight. Also, try to include a variety in your diet. This will ensure a more balanced diet.

Exercise. Regular exercise can help you to lose weight and improve your mood. You can stop eating emotional food and engage in physical activity. It will improve both your mind and overall well-being. For advice about what the best exercise routine is for you, it's a good idea to consult with your physician. This is especially important for overweight people. Perhaps you can start by walking for 20 minutes. This will help to burn calories and improve your heart health.

Do not eat out of boredom. Instead of eating out of boredom, try replacing this bad habit with something that is fun and enjoyable. It will be much easier to eat less when you're engaged in a relaxing pastime. If you don't feel like walking by yourself, consider getting a dog you can walk with. Your dog will notify you when it is time for you to go for a walk. Dogs can be an excellent friend and motivator for going outside to walk.

Get enough good sleep. There are many benefits to making sure you get enough sleep each night. Do not eat large quantities of food if your energy is low or you feel exhausted. You won't get any energy boost from binging. Don't eat large amounts before you go bed. This could lead to heartburn, insomnia, and weight gain.

Limit your exposures to tempting foods. If binge eating is a problem, and you keep your favourite foods close at hand, it will make it more difficult for you to get over it. It is better to eliminate unhealthy foods entirely from your home or to keep them in sealed containers. Schedule the intake of special treats foods in your meal planner to control your eating habits.

Maintain healthy eating habits. It is crucial not to skip meals. Avoiding meals will lead to binging episodes later in your day. Make sure you have three healthy meals per week, with healthy snacks in between. It is a good idea to have a large breakfast to begin the day. A good breakfast will reduce the amount of calories you consume later in your day. Talk to your doctor about taking vitamin and mineral supplements.

Keep track of what you eat with a Food Journal. For those who suffer from binge eating disorder, it is important to keep track of their food intake. It is vital to be able to record how much, which food, and what their mood was while eating. You can keep a journal to track what food a person eats and what mood they are in when they have a binge. It is a valuable resource to keep track of during therapy sessions as well as for routine check-ups.

Improve your body image. One reason for binge-eating disorder is low self-esteem. Learn how to improve your body image for those who binge. But this doesn't mean that they need to dress up in order to impress their friends. It's more about making them feel good about their appearance.

You can make yourself feel better by pampering yourself regularly. They could go for a massage or buy a new dress. You should encourage anything that improves your self-esteem.

Offer reassuring assistance. People suffering from bingeing need the support and encouragement they can get from their loved ones and support groups, especially when it comes to the emotional side. It is possible to gain support by having a meaningful conversation with someone who cares enough. This is true even for those who aren't professional health professionals, but they must be accepting and not judgmental. A person suffering from binge eating should be supported by loved ones who will show that they won't judge them in any way.

It is essential to follow the treatment program in order for your success. A treatment program should not be broken by binge-eaters. It won't help them if their therapy sessions and support groups are missed without valid reasons. They should make sure they take their medications as directed and not skip them.

They must fully commit to following a weight loss plan. If they do make mistakes on the journey to complete recovery from binge eating they should not be discouraged. Instead, pick yourself up and keep moving forward. It is possible to stop eating bingeing by persevering with your efforts and not giving up.

www.ingramcontent.com/pod-product-compliance
Lightning Source LLC
Chambersburg PA
CBHW050401120526
44590CB00015B/1772